Patients increasingly turn to resources such as the Internet and texts written for the "lay person" to understand various treatment approaches for back pain. In *Back Pain Understood: A Cutting-Edge Approach To Healing Your Back*, Dr. Hainline has given us a comprehensive and excellent resource in an easy to understand format. Dr. Hainline not only describes the painful anatomic abnormalities of back pain, but also emphasizes the often-overlooked "mind-body" connection. He eloquently distinguishes the need for non-operative and operative care of back pain. This book is an invaluable guide to help patients make informed decisions regarding their treatment options, and is a must read for patients with back and spinal problems.

—*Andrew C. Hecht, MD*
Chief Orthopaedic Spine Surgery
Mt Sinai Medical Center
and School of Medicine

Back pain is a bane for most physicians to manage properly, and any mismanagement can completely undermine the aspirations and functioning of the patient—ranging from the elite athlete to the sedentary worker. Dr. Hainline has written a comprehensive, pragmatic and compassionate book that expertly navigates patients, physicians and clinicians alike. He blends science, clinical excellence and wisdom to create a refreshing, wholistic medical approach to diagnosing and treating low back pain. I highly recommend this book to anyone interested in this subject.

—*Elliot Pellman, MD*
Medical Liaison, National Football League
Medical Advisor, Major League Baseball

I have worked with Dr. Hainline in the world of professional tennis for over 10 years. He is a highly educated and thoughtful individual who is willing to think outside the box. Many healthcare professionals have a narrow-minded way of diagnosing and managing back pain and back injuries. Dr. Hainline gives us an informative and refreshingly new way to address back pair · · ·us to be open-minded to the many different treatment lt problem.

D1403121

—*Doug Spreen ATC*
Trainer for Andy Roddick
·ainer, US Davis Cup Team

Back Pain Understood

A Cutting-Edge Approach
To Healing Your Back

Brian Hainline, MD

Medicus Press

Library of Congress Control Number: 2006938763

ISBN-13: 978-0-9787727-0-3
ISBN   0-9787727-0-9

This publication is designed to provide accurate and authoritative information in regard to the subject matter covered. It is sold with the understanding that neither the author nor the publisher shall be liable or responsible for any loss, injury or damage allegedly arising from any information or suggestion in this book. The treatments, medicines, procedures and other suggestions contained in this book are not intended as a substitute for consulting with a physician. The reader should consult with a physician in matters relating to her/his health and particularly with respect to any symptoms that may require diagnosis or medical attention.

First Printing

To order visit www.medicuspress.com and/or
www.backpainunderstood.com

Cover design by Editora Novo Art
Cover photograph by © Deborah Kuzniecky

To Orrin and Caron—
In thanks for encouraging me
To see with my heart
And to write as I see

Contents

Introduction

While traveling with my family in Western Africa, I was given the opportunity to meet with the local medicine man in Korogo, Ivory Coast. I felt privileged to listen to a man revered for his wisdom, practicality, and compassion. The agreement to meet came through a series of intermediaries, and he asked beforehand that I bring antimalarial and antidiarrheal medications. He wished to hear me speak about these medications—their origin, their mode of action—and he planned to utilize them along with his own botanical remedies. The reality of today's medicine presents itself in many forms. Whereas I understood the chemical and pharmacologic properties of the antimalarial drug mefloquine, I had no idea of its unique source in Mother Nature.

The medicine man viewed life as a constant interplay between humans and nature. His role was as a mediator between the afflicted human and the remedies provided by nature. Most medical conditions were infectious in nature, which he could treat effectively with natural botanical mixtures and the proper dose of rest.

As we embraced the eternal day, graced by each other's presence and the shade of a tree centuries old, the village slowly gathered about this sacred space. The overall setting was pure and primitive relative to our technological, scatological standards. And yet, what seemed to reign here was an ordained sense of order. Mud huts were immaculately clean. Gums were healthy as teeth yellowed naturally with age. The local water was toxic to my pristine, naïve stomach, yet quenched the thirst of the village in need. Everyone had their place, including the gods. Life was simple, in a complex circular hierarchy involving the masters, the elders, the mothers, the children, the land, the gods, and one's allegiance to order.

I asked the medicine man about pain, and his answer shocked me into opening my eyes to the village around me. Here, pain served a useful, singular purpose. When a worker became injured, he or she experienced pain with the injury. Pain subsided as the injury healed. The medicine man knew of low back pain and disc herniation, and this, too, he expressed as a short-lived companion of injury. As we went further into our discussion of pain, we seemed to be lost in translation when it came to chronic pain. The villagers too, looked confused as I conjured up images to describe this debilitating and familiar disease. It was eventually understood that the concept of a chronic pain syndrome was not merely untranslatable, but incomprehensible.

Although malaria flirts with the villagers of Korogo, chronic pain afflicts more than 60 million Americans. And, although our Western world has seemingly conquered malaria, we are constantly reminded that our dance with life is filled with other afflictions. But why chronic pain—so much of which is chronic low back pain? To answer this question, we must step back and reanalyze our understanding of pain and our understanding of our own dance with life, our dance within our society.

The medicine man looked at me with frank eyes and asked, "But why would pain persist for months or years in someone? I have never seen this, nor have my teachers, through generations, ever spoken of such a human condition."

In this book I will try to answer the medicine man's question. I can only do so from my perspective as a Western-trained physician and as one who listens, day in and day out, to patients from America and other parts of the Western world. This is my conceptual framework, one that I trust is commonplace with you, the reader. Specifically, I hope to bring an understanding of low back pain to light, a malady whose ubiquity and chronicity shapes the destiny of our home, workplace, and medical office.

We have no universally accepted understanding of low back pain in its myriad presentations. Nor do we have a universal approach to management. Chiropractors, acupuncturists, orthopedic surgeons, neurosurgeons, rheumatologists, neurologists, osteopaths, physiatrists, nurses, physician assistants, massage therapists, physical therapists, athletic trainers, kinesiologists, homeopaths, naturopaths, primary care physicians, neighbors, friends, relatives—all have an opinion of proper diagnosis and management. Many overlap, and many diverge. Although I cannot assume to have a unifying answer for all, this book is an attempt to find common ground among the seeming disarray of low back pain world views.

We begin with a discussion of pain. We must try to understand pain not simply as an anatomic focus, but also as a physiological expression within an individual person. Yes, low back pain may arise from a herniated disc, but the intensity or chronicity of low back pain may be influenced by the faulty biomechanics of the disc segment as much as by the fear, apprehension, rage, or sadness of the individual carrying the disc. Pain is multifaceted, and serves to warn as well as to reveal. Emotions—like pain itself—have their physical expression. As we keep this in mind, we may appreciate the meaning of chronic pain, and discover more about the human soul as it works in tandem with the body.

We move from a discussion of pain to an overview of the anatomy and physiology of the lower back. From there, we delve into the diversity of management approaches to low back pain, and we then analyze various low back pain syndromes. The anatomic and physiologic conceptual framework of our discussion spring from the mind of modern medicine. I blend this conceptual framework with the richness of anecdotes and stories of healing, because these provide the fertile ground for teaching, comprehending, and bridging science with the human heart.

Acknowledgments

I am indebted to so many people who helped me to bring my ideas about back pain to a finished book of labor and love. Steve Pacia gave me the opportunity and format to write this book, and his colleagues at Medicus Press—Yvonne Zelenka, Joann Woy and Patricia Wallenburg—provided expert assistance at every step of the way. Clotilde and Arthur Hainline helped transform a rough draft into a spirit-filled and cohesive text. Kathy Gorham, nurse practitioner extraordinaire, used her red pen to bring consistent logic to my writing. Maura Flynn combined skill with imagination in her drawings, and she recognized where additional photographs and illustrations would be helpful. Dan Goldman brought life to my explanations with his photographer's eye. Kathleen Finzel poured over multiple imaging studies that matched the clinical syndromes.

In this day and age of physician weariness from managed care, I feel blessed to awaken with a passion for my profession. As a physician, we have the sacred opportunity to combine wisdom and genuine concern as we hold the health of another human being in our care. My passion flourishes in part because of my work environment. ProHEALTH Care Associates is a multi-specialty group with over 100 medical providers; our CEO, David Cooper, is unwavering in his vision and commitment to outstanding medical care. Within the Division of Neurology and Integrative Pain Medicine, Danielle Beltran brings order to life in her role as office manager, and my two associate directors—Dan Brietstein and Caron Hunter—represent the yin and yang of comprehensive and compassionate integrative pain medicine. It is within this framework that I care for patients with back pain, and this caring has become the fertile soil for my book.

I am forever grateful to my family. Pascale, Clotilde, Arthur, and Juliette—you nourish my creative energy and daily discipline, and you bring meaning and purpose to my being.

Overview of Low Back Pain

CHAPTER 1

Types of Pain

NOCICEPTIVE PAIN

Pain is a universal experience. If you place your hand over fire, your hand will immediately withdraw, and you will simultaneously experience pain. This is because receptors in your skin identify factors in the environment that may cause damage to your body. In the case of the fire, the heat can lead to tissue destruction, because your skin can only tolerate temperatures to a certain degree. Thus, in this case, the pain serves a useful, protective purpose, and this type of pain is known medically as nociceptive pain.

Different types of pain receptors exist, formally called *nociceptors*. When nociceptors cause a pain response following activation, we call this nociceptive pain. Mechanical, chemical, and temperature-sensitive nociceptors exist. If these receptors are stimulated in such a way that a critical threshold is surpassed, then the body responds by sending a pain signal. Very often, this pain signal is coupled with a reflex withdrawal action by the appropriate body part (Figure 1.1).

Nociceptors are found throughout the body, including in the skin, muscles, joints, and organs. Although they do serve a very useful, protective purpose, they are not the sole cause of pain, and this is a recurring theme throughout the book.

One of the unfortunate mistakes of pain management is the belief that chronic pain is caused by activation of nociceptors. Patients may have longstanding pain, and it has become indoctrinated in our society that, if someone has pain, a singular anatomic explanation must exist for the pain. This leads to the mistaken notion that, if we can simply block or correct the apparent anatomic nociceptive basis of pain, then the pain will be relieved. The multitude of failed back surgeries (spinal surgery that does not alleviate back pain) and failed spinal injections (spinal injections

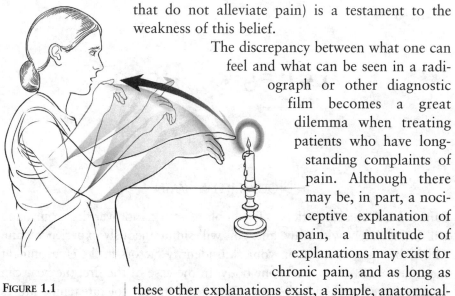

FIGURE 1.1
Reflex withdrawal from a painful stimulus.

that do not alleviate pain) is a testament to the weakness of this belief.

The discrepancy between what one can feel and what can be seen in a radiograph or other diagnostic film becomes a great dilemma when treating patients who have long-standing complaints of pain. Although there may be, in part, a nociceptive explanation of pain, a multitude of explanations may exist for chronic pain, and as long as these other explanations exist, a simple, anatomically directed treatment plan will be ineffective. This point leads to a discussion of other types of pain.

NEUROPATHIC PAIN

The nervous system includes the brain, spinal cord, and peripheral nerves (the nerves outside the spinal cord). In a simplistic scheme, the peripheral nerves constantly provide signals that are relayed through the spinal cord to the brain. The brain interprets these signals and then sends a response back down to the spine and through the peripheral nerves. For example, if the finger is suddenly exposed to an extremely hot temperature, the peripheral nerve sends a signal to the spinal cord and to the brain. The brain immediately sends a signal of pain, while also directing an immediate withdrawal movement away from the heat source. This withdrawal movement is not even under conscious control, and the pain is appropriate to the injury or inciting event, which means it is nociceptive pain (Figure 1.2).

Neuropathic pain is pain that persists at least 1 month longer than one might reasonably expect following an inciting or noxious event. As in the example above, when you burn your finger, you normally experience pain, but within hours to days, the pain normally subsides. If healing is prolonged, for example because of an infection, and pain therefore persists longer, the ongoing pain response remains appropriate to an inciting event, in this case the infection.

On the other hand, you can burn your finger and, although the burn wound may heal completely and uneventfully, the pain may persist and become transformed, possibly lasting for months or even years. This prolonged or transformed pain is neuropathic pain.

A classic example of prolonged, neuropathic pain is the severe back pain that persists even after a patient has undergone seemingly perfect spinal fusion surgery. Even if the surgery is "perfect" from a mechanical and spinal fusion point of view, the pain persists. From the spine surgeon's point of view, the fusion is solid, and the pain must be the result of some other cause. The patient can be made to feel that he is the cause of the pain. But from the patient's point of view, because the spinal surgery has failed, the surgeon must be in the wrong, and the faulty 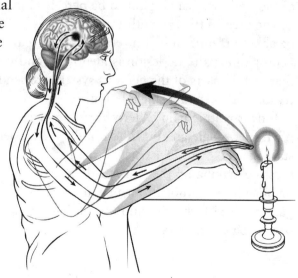 back must be the cause of pain. The disconnect between the surgeon and patient can leave the patient

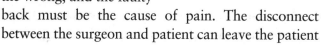

FIGURE 1.2
Brain response following a painful stimulus.

5

feeling desperate. The patient is experiencing subjective pain and there is no way to prove by objective criteria what is causing the pain.

Certain diseases and conditions have been well described as causing neuropathic pain. In all cases of neuropathic pain, there exists a lesion or dysfunction of the nervous system that causes the pain. A *lesion* is any change in the body's normal anatomy, and it can range from a small scar to a large tumor. For example, multiple sclerosis (MS)—an autoimmune disease—can sometimes cause a lesion in one of the nerves that controls sensation in the face. This nerve—the trigeminal nerve—normally allows perception of touch to the face. If a strategically located MS plaque exists in a key pathway of the trigeminal nerve, this can lead to a prolonged facial pain. As opposed to nociceptive pain, this prolonged pain can last for weeks, months, or even years. Thus, the pain can no longer be called nociceptive or protective. The pain is caused by a lesion of the nervous system.

Interestingly, neuropathic pain does not arise necessarily from a lesion, but can result from dysfunction of the nervous system. This leads to one of the most heated areas of debate within pain-management circles. Our Western culture thrives on defining various circumstances in a linear, cause-and-effect manner. Using this type of thinking, a lesion in one part of the brain will cause pain to be perceived in one part of the body.

The great difficulty with the word "dysfunction" is that one may not be able to identify a lesion responsible for pain. Indeed, in many cases of neuropathic pain, no lesion is identified, and we must rather hypothesize that certain parts of the nervous system are sending signals aberrantly for reasons other than a single lesion.

If neuropathic pain is derived from a dysfunctional state, and not simply from a single anatomic lesion, the inexperienced clinician may simply state that no "cause" exists for the pain, thus suggesting that the patient must be making up the pain, or that the pain is somehow psychosomatic or imaginary. Although an unequivocal psychological component to all pain does exist, this does not mean that physical pain has been incited by psychological distress.

ACUTE PAIN

Acute pain is pain that is short-lived. Acute pain is a universal sensation and again, we move back to the example of placing one's finger over a flame. The pain is immediate, and it resolves quickly. Thus, acute pain is usually nociceptive.

Another example of acute pain is lumbar strain. Lifting something quite heavy can lead to a sudden muscle pull, then a sudden experience of low back pain. The pain may last for hours or days, depending on the severity of the lumbar strain. The pain is appropriate: The nerves in the lumbar support muscles detect a mechanical disruption in muscle fibers and send signals that result in the perception of pain in the low back. The pain is also protective and relatively short-lived. Generally speaking, acute pain results from sudden activation of nociceptors, and that source of pain can be traced to an injury or potential injury affecting a specific part of the body.

CHRONIC PAIN

Chronic pain persists for at least 1 month longer than one might reasonably expect following an inciting or noxious event. Chronic pain and neuropathic pain are interchangeable terms. Chronic pain generally is associated with a multitude of other factors, because the pain becomes intertwined with all aspects of the patient's life. Often, patients who experience chronic pain suffer physically, emotionally, mentally, socially, nutritionally, and spiritually. Indeed, the term *chronic pain syndrome* means that a patient's life has become defined by pain in all spheres of his existence.

PAIN AND EMOTION

Pain is defined by the International Association for the Study of Pain as "an unpleasant sensory and emotional experience associated with actual or potential tissue damage, or described in terms of such damage." From this definition, we can see that pain is not a simple sensory experience. An emotion always is associated with that pain. The emotional response may range from mild unpleasantness to incredible fear and panic. When we analyze the pathways that are responsible for the perception of pain, we come to understand that many areas of the brain that normally subserve emotions are intimately related to pain perception.

The familiar wartime story of a soldier developing a severe injury, yet not perceiving any pain for some time thereafter because his life is in imminent danger, is a classic example of how emotions can influence pain. In this case, the complex relationship between the signals indicating tissue damage, and the threat to the person's life otherwise, lead to no immediate experience of pain. Once the danger has passed, the appropriate pain response is experienced.

Whereas a life-threatening fear response can delay perception of pain, other emotions can augment the pain experience. Depression is a universal component of chronic pain. It is difficult if not impossible to completely alleviate chronic pain if depression persists. The depression leads to a *sensitization* of the nervous system, which means that pain perception becomes augmented.

A patient with post-traumatic stress disorder, or a patient who has experienced profound stress experiences at some point in his life, may be more vulnerable to neuropathic pain. Sometimes, an injury or potential injury leads to a nonconscious recognition of a link between the potential or actual injury and prior traumatic experience. The nervous system pathways from the prior traumatic experience can become intermingled with the more recent tissue injury pathways, the nervous system becomes sensitized, and the pain expression becomes exaggerated. In some cases, a new circuitry develops in which the anxiety pathways are so commingled with the pain pathways that the pain pathway becomes constantly activated, leading to the experience of chronic pain.

In all these examples, the patient is not consciously causing pain or causing a lack of perception of pain. Rather, the nervous system is responding in a way that is unique to that patient's experience. This becomes one of the most difficult aspects of treating patients who have chronic pain. The clinician must try to understand the patient's unique circumstances, and the patient must be open to sharing and exploring his unique circumstances with the clinician.

SUMMARY POINTS

- Nociceptive pain is pain that is appropriate to an injury or inciting event. This pain is short-lived.
- Neuropathic pain and chronic pain are interchangeable terms. Both mean that pain persists 1 month longer than what one might expect from an injury or inciting event.

- Neuropathic pain can be caused either by a lesion within the nervous system or by dysfunction of the nervous system.
- Chronic pain and emotions can intermingle in such a way that the individual's experience of pain becomes more prolonged and more severe.
- Chronic pain is not a psychosomatic condition. Rather, it is the result of the nervous system responding to a unique set of individual experiences.

CHAPTER 2

Low Back Anatomy

The anatomy of the low back consists of the bones of the spine (vertebrae); the discs between these bones; the bones of the pelvis; and muscles, ligaments, tendons, and nerves. This chapter provides a general overview of essential aspects of low back anatomy.

THE SPINAL COLUMN

The spinal column is the deepest layer of the spine and is composed of the vertebral body, the discs between each vertebral body, and the muscles, tendons, and nerves that form a complex web around the vertebral body. Normally, there are seven cervical, twelve thoracic, and five lumbar vertebrae. The *cervical vertebrae* comprise the neck region. The *thoracic vertebrae* comprise the mid back region. The *lumbar vertebrae* comprise the low back region (Figure 2.1).

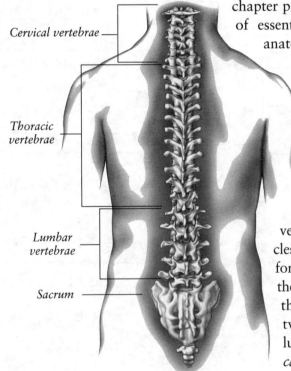

Cervical vertebrae

Thoracic vertebrae

Lumbar vertebrae

Sacrum

FIGURE 2.1A
A back view of the spinal column.

We can think of the spinal vertebrae as forming a continuum of 25 individual bones, with pairs of vertebrae forming a spinal joint. Thus, within the lumbar spine, the first lumbar vertebrae and the second lumbar vertebrae form a joint, the second and third lumbar vertebrae are a spinal joint, and so on. Each joint is responsible for allowing a certain type of movement. In the lumbar spine, the greatest degree of movement occurs between the two lowest lumbar joints (Figure 2.2).

The spinal joint can be divided into an anterior (closer to the belly) or weight-bearing segment and a posterior (closer to the back) or non–weight-bearing segment. The

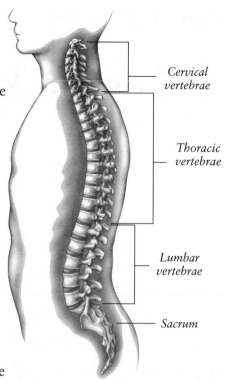

Cervical vertebrae

Thoracic vertebrae

Lumbar vertebrae

Sacrum

FIGURE 2.1B
A side view of the spinal column.

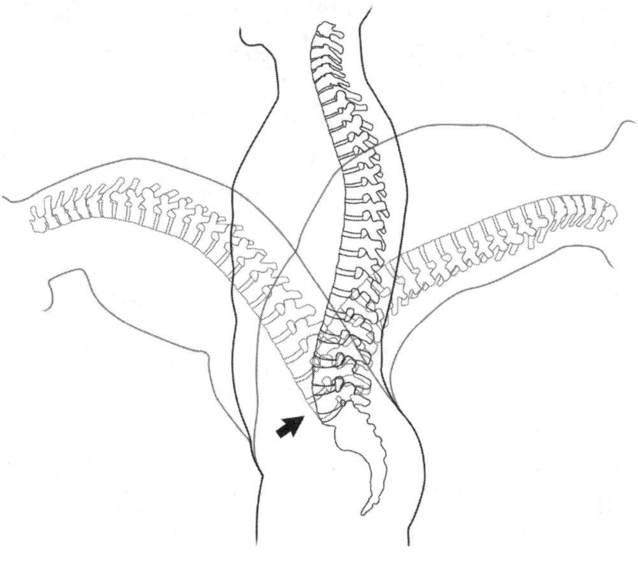

FIGURE 2.2
Spinal movement in the low lumbar spine.

11

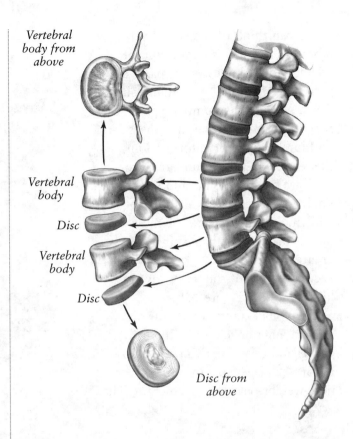

FIGURE 2.3
Details of the spinal joint complex.

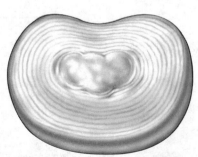

FIGURE 2.4
The lumbar disc.

weight-bearing segment of the spinal joint is comprised of the two large cylindrical-shaped vertebral bodies, with a lumbar disc in between (Figure 2.3).

The lumbar disc provides both stability and mobility to the lumbar spine. The lumbar disc has an outer *annulus*, which is a firm, fibroelastic mesh. The inner part of the disc is called the *nucleus*, and this is essentially a proteinaceous gel (Figure 2.4).

Until about the third decade of life, the inner nucleus is approximately 90% water. Over time, the water content of the disc gradually diminishes. When the disc is healthy with abundant water, compression of the

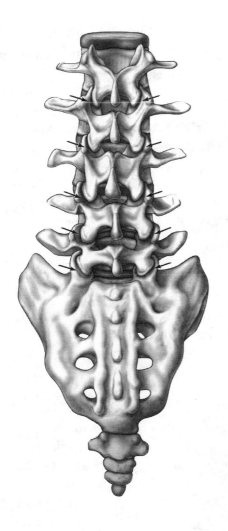

FIGURE 2.5
Back view demonstrating (arrows) the facet joints.

spinal joint is possible, and stability of movement is more assured.

The posterior part of the spine allows spinal movement via the *facets*. The facets, sometimes called the facet joints, are normally smooth, gliding joints that allow the spine to move in a front and back type of motion or a sideways motion, or a combination thereof, depending on their orientation. In the lumbar spine, the facets allow trunk flexion and extension movements (Figure 2.5).

13

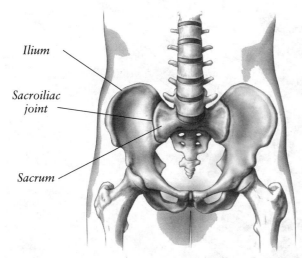

Ilium

Sacroiliac
joint

Sacrum

FIGURE 2.6
*Front view of the
sacrum and
sacroiliac joint.*

The lumbar spine is connected to the *sacrum*. The sacrum is a large triangular bone that lies just inferior to (below) the lumbar spine. The sacrum also connects to the iliac bone, which forms part of the pelvis, by way of the *sacroiliac joint* (Figure 2.6). This is a relatively thin and immobile joint. During pregnancy, the sacroiliac joint actually enlarges somewhat, to help promote increased mobility during delivery.

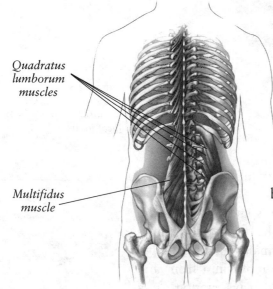

Quadratus
lumborum
muscles

Multifidus
muscle

FIGURE 2.7
*Back view of the deep
muscles of the
low back.*

LOW BACK MUSCULATURE

Key muscles attach not only to the lumbar spine, but also to the ribs and the pelvis, which interconnect from the pelvis to the neck region. Two deep muscle groups in the lower back are the *multifidus* and the *quadratus lumborum* (Figure 2.7). It is difficult to feel these muscles by touching the body, but a skilled clinician, while performing manual work such as physical therapy, can feel when these muscles are contracting normally or abnormally. In addition, various imaging techniques can delineate if these muscles appear normal, or if they have developed an atrophied (shrunken) appearance. These deep-layer muscles are critical for day-to-day movement and spine stability.

Another important deep muscle is called the *psoas muscle*. Very often, the psoas is referred to as the iliopsoas, which is really a combination of two muscle groups—the iliacus and the psoas. These muscles connect the lumbar spine to the hip flexors (Figure 2.8). When the iliopsoas is contracting improperly—from a chronic strain, for example—spinal movement can be impacted negatively.

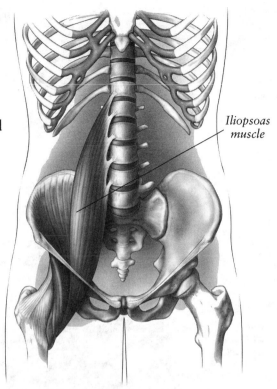

Iliopsoas muscle

FIGURE 2.8
Front view of the iliopsoas muscle.

In patients with chronic pain, these deep muscle groups commonly malfunction. They may be the primary source of pain, or they may be an integral maladaptive response to chronic pain. For example, chronic iliopsoas strain is an underdiagnosed cause of chronic low back pain. However, a patient with a progressively degenerative lumbar spine also may have concomitant iliopsoas muscles contracting abnormally on a chronic basis, thus helping to perpetuate the cycle of malfunction and pain.

In patients who experience chronic low back pain, it is fairly common for these deep muscle groups to malfunction, but unfortunately, these are often overlooked in pain management. Simply per-

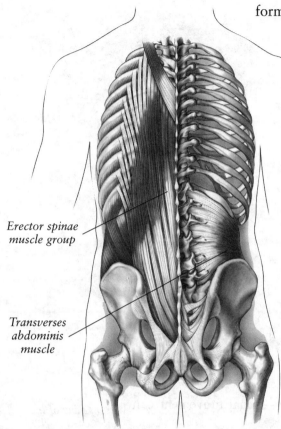

Erector spinae
muscle group

Transverses
abdominis
muscle

Figure 2.9
*Back view of the
erector spinae
muscles.*

forming spinal surgery, or providing spinal injections, is not a sufficient answer for a patient who suffers with chronic back pain from maladaptation of these deep muscle groups.

The *erector spinae* comprise the outer layer of back muscles. The erector spinae muscles can be palpated (touched) easily. In acute lumbar strain, you often can see and palpate the spasm of the erector spinae muscle groups (Figure 2.9).

Complementing the back muscles are the abdominal muscles, which include the *transverses abdominis, external oblique, internal oblique,* and *rectus abdominis* muscles. These muscle groups become activated in day-to-day flexion and rotation of the spine, and they perform a constant balancing act with the low back muscles (Figure 2.10).

Pain-Sensitive Structures

Essentially, all aspects of the lower back, ranging from the deep spinal joint to the outer spinal muscles, are innervated by pain-sensitive nerves. If tissue injury suddenly develops at any level of the spinal joint or muscles, the pain-sensitive structures—com-

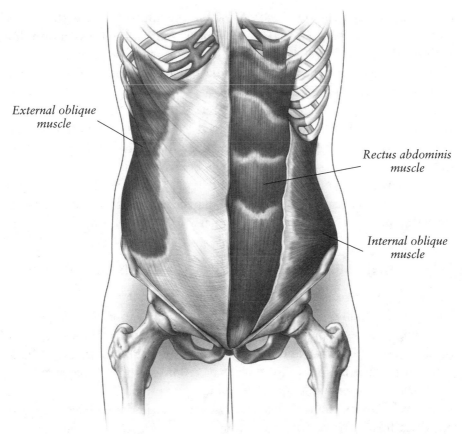

External oblique
muscle

Rectus abdominis
muscle

Internal oblique
muscle

prised of nociceptors—become activated, and pain can be perceived. However, this does not mean that an abnormality within the lower back will necessarily cause pain. This is another extremely important point when trying to understand patients who suffer with chronic pain: Anatomic lesions do not necessarily equate with pain.

Because imaging studies are now readily available in our Western culture, we can analyze the anatomy of the lumbar spine in ways that were not previously possible. As will be discussed later, magnetic resonance imaging (MRI) is a sensitive tool that is used to assess the structure of the lumbar spine. Numerous studies have demonstrated that patients

FIGURE 2.10
Front view of the abdominal muscles.

can have ruptured and degenerated discs in the lumbar spine without ever having developed pain. Indeed, a spinal nerve can be compressed by a disc without the patient ever having suffered pain at the level of that nerve. Thus, the dilemma occurs when sorting out the meaning of an imaging abnormality within the lumbar spine.

As a corollary, an imaging study may reveal that the lumbar spine appears completely normal, yet the patient may have excruciating low back pain. The absence of a well-defined anatomic lesion does not mean that the patient cannot have pain. Rather, the pain may stem from some other type of dysfunction within the nervous system. Ultimately, the experienced clinician must determine the source of pain. The source may be from irritation of a pain-sensitive structure, from dysfunction of the nervous system elsewhere, or both.

ANATOMIC VERSUS PHYSIOLOGIC BASIS OF PAIN

One of the most confusing concepts in diagnosing and managing patients with pain is to differentiate between an anatomic cause of pain versus a physiologic cause of pain. Many times, the *etiology* or cause of pain is a combination of anatomy and physiology. It is important to grasp this basic concept, because failure to do so leads to failure in pain management.

As a simplistic example of an anatomic cause of pain, consider someone who develops a ruptured lumbar disc. As we discussed previously, the lumbar discs form part of the spinal joint, and they are the stabilizing and shock-absorbing structures between the lumbar vertebra. If a lumbar disc suddenly tears, and its inner contents rupture, the ruptured content can exert pressure on a nerve. Commonly, the nerve affected forms part of the large sciatic nerve in the leg, and pain is perceived in the affected leg. Patients with acute lumbar disc herniation that compresses a lumbar nerve generally have a classic presentation: They develop low back pain that radiates into the buttock and down the leg. This is known as *sciatica*.

In assessing such a patient, a clinician can discern the level of the lumbar spine affected as well as the nerve root affected. An MRI or other imaging study can detect with certainty the disc affected, and it can demonstrate the pressure of the rupture disc on the nerve. We can state with confidence that the anatomic cause of the pain in this particular example is the ruptured disc compressing the lumbar nerve root, leading to pain in the distribution of the nerve root.

As an example of a physiologically based pain, consider the patient who develops low back pain across the entire lower back, which persists for months. Pain is present regardless of the patient's body position. The patient is diagnosed with *myofascial pain* (discussed in Chapter 15), and the patient is told that a herniated disc or a pinched nerve is not responsible for the pain.

The patient may become upset in learning that no simple explanation exists for the pain. Alternatively, the clinician may fail to understand how severe this pain may be, and may state simply that the pain is "in your head." Although we may want to state that myofascial pain has a simple anatomic explanation, such pain is mediated, rather, by an alteration in the nervous system's processing of pain signals. In many ways, myofascial pain is like migraine: Certain pain pathways within the nervous system become hypersensitive and begin to fire on a regular basis, even though no structural problem or nociceptive signal indicates tissue damage or potential tissue damage.

In the case of the ruptured herniated disc, treatment should be focused on the biomechanics of the disc. In the case of myofascial pain, treatment should be focused on trying to understand how to help change the body's physiology.

Even in the above two examples, no clear separation is present between anatomy and physiology. Some patients may have prolonged sciatica-like pain even as the ruptured disc material has begun to resorb and is no longer placing pressure on the nerve root. With myofascial pain, several muscular maladaptations may need to be addressed physically. Understanding that pain is driven by a combination of anatomy and physiology becomes the cornerstone of effective pain management.

Summary Points

- The spinal column is comprised of vertebral bodies, discs, muscles, nerves, tendons, and ligaments. Spinal vertebrae pair as two-level joints that allow for movement.
- The lumbar disc is important for providing both stability and mobility.
- The muscles around the lumbar spine must function in a well-coordinated manner. They frequently malfunction following spinal injury, or as part of a cycle of chronic pain.

■ Sometimes, pain is clearly related to an anatomic problem within the spinal column. Other times, pain originates from a change in the body's physiology, even with normal spinal anatomy.

■ It is common for lumbar discs to degenerate or even to herniate without necessarily causing pain.

CHAPTER 3

Clinicians Who Treat Low Back Pain

A wide variety of physicians and health care practitioners may diagnose and manage patients suffering with low back pain, and they represent a multitude of disciplines and conceptual frameworks. For example, a pain anesthesiologist who specializes in providing injections into the spine has a much different point of reference than does a chiropractor, who specializes in spinal manipulation. Pain anesthesiologists and chiropractors may work in a complementary manner, however, and may even be part of the same multidisciplinary team. Yet, they are more often worlds apart, both from a treatment and communication perspective.

This chapter provides a broad overview of clinicians who diagnose and manage patients with low back pain. This serves as a useful reference point when discussing specific low back pain conditions.

PHYSICIANS

Physicians are medical doctors or osteopathic doctors who have completed an accredited medical school or osteopathic medical school. Following successful completion of such schooling, physicians then undergo further training, which is a combination of an internship and a residency. Such training allows the physician to specialize in one or more areas of practice, ranging from family practice medicine to a surgical subspecialty. Generally speaking, physicians have admitting privileges to hospitals. Physicians who have successfully completed medical school have the degree M.D. (Medical Doctor) following their names. Physicians who have successfully completed an osteopathic school of medicine have the initials D.O. (Doctor of Osteopathy) after their names. Although a medical doctor and an osteopathic doctor may be indistinguishable in their day-to-day practice, some doctors of osteopathy practice medicine with much more of a focus on the spine as the center of medical health. Such doctors utilize spinal manipulation as an essential component of their day-to-day practice.

Anesthesiologist

An anesthesiologist is a physician who specializes in providing anesthesia to patients who are to undergo surgical procedures. A subspecialty of anesthesia that pertains to patients with low back pain is called *pain anesthesiology*. Anesthesiologists who specialize in pain anesthesiology have completed additional training in pain medicine. This training includes a specialty focus on diagnosing and managing various spinal and peripheral nerve conditions. Pain anesthesiologists typically work by providing pain medications and by delivering therapeutic injections. Pain anesthesiologists often work as part of a multispecialty pain medicine group.

Family Medicine Physician

Family medicine physicians specialize in primary health care, and such physicians are often the first line of management for a wide variety of medical conditions, including pediatrics, adult medical care, geriatrics, and gynecologic care. For example, a family medicine physician may be the first person to diagnose a patient with high blood pressure or diabetes and, depending on how complicated the case is, can manage the patient or may in turn refer the patient to a specialist. Because low back pain is commonplace, the family medicine physician is often the first person to encounter a patient with this problem. Typically, the physician then prescribes medication or makes a referral to a physical therapist or chiropractor.

Internist

An internist is a physician who specializes in adult general medical care. An internist receives specialty training in a wide variety of adult medical conditions and usually serves as the primary care physician for the patient. Most general medical problems are managed by internists, and more complex problems are referred to specialists. As with family medicine physicians, internists are often the first point of management for a patient who is suffering with low back pain. The internist may provide medication, give a prescription for physical therapy, or make a referral to another health care provider.

Neurologist

A neurologist is a physician who specializes in diagnosing and managing diseases and conditions of the nervous system, which includes the brain, spinal cord, peripheral nerves, and muscles. Prototypic neurologic conditions include multiple sclerosis, Parkinson's disease, epilepsy, and stroke. Some neurologists have a special interest in disorders of the spine, but this is not universally true. Very often, a neurologist is asked to see a patient when the possibility exists for a compressed nerve, nerve damage, or spinal cord damage as it relates to a low back or spinal condition. Thus, a neurologist may simply make a diagnosis and report back to the referring physician regarding the presence of nerve damage, and this should help to determine future management. Other neurologists are more hands-on, and will manage all aspects of the patient's low back condition.

Neurosurgeon

A neurosurgeon is a physician who specializes in the surgical treatment of nervous system disorders. Prototypic neurosurgical interventions include surgery for tumors of the brain and spine or repair of a ruptured aneurysm. Some neurosurgeons have received specialty training in spine surgery. It should not be assumed that all neurosurgeons treat spinal conditions, because some have little interest or training in disorders of the spine. It also should not be assumed that if spinal surgery is necessary, then a neurosurgeon is the most qualified person to do such surgery. In essence, both neurosurgeons and orthopedic surgeons can receive very similar subspecialty training in spinal surgery. If a patient has a tumor of the spine, a neurosurgeon is the most appropriate person to perform such surgery. However, for more common spinal conditions, such as a herniated lumbar disc or spinal stenosis, either a qualified neurosurgeon or orthopedic surgeon can perform surgery.

Orthopedic Surgeon

An orthopedic surgeon is a physician who specializes in diagnosing, managing, and performing surgery for disorders and conditions of the bones. Prototypic orthopedic surgical intervention is management of bone fractures. Some orthopedic surgeons are generalists and manage all types of musculoskeletal problems. Others are specialists and only manage conditions within their field of subspecialty, for example treating knee or shoulder conditions. Not all orthopedic surgeons are adept at treating spinal conditions. Some manage spinal conditions nonoperatively, and others specialize in surgery of the spine. As with neurosurgeons, some orthopedic surgeons receive subspecialty training in spinal surgery. Such orthopedic surgeons work within a network of clinicians who manage low back pain from both a nonsurgical and surgical viewpoint.

Pain Medicine Specialist

Pain medicine is a relatively new subspecialty. Whereas, several years ago, any physician could state that he practiced pain management, now board certification procedures are in place for pain medicine. To receive board certification, a licensed physician must take specialty training in pain medicine, which focuses on medication management and therapeutic injections for patients with various chronic pain conditions. Anesthesiologists were the first physicians to develop a specialty board for pain medicine. Now neurologists, internists, physiatrists, and orthopedic surgeons also can become subspecialized in pain medicine. Pain medicine specialists often manage patients with chronic low back pain and other chronic pain conditions.

Physiatrist

A physiatrist is a doctor who specializes in physical rehabilitation. Physiatrists receive general medical training, then specialty training in rehabilitating patients with handicapping neurologic or orthopedic conditions. Such conditions include, but are not limited to, stroke, amputations, and spinal injuries. Many physiatrists have a special interest in treating disorders of the spine, and they also have received training in providing therapeutic injections into the spinal region.

Psychiatrist

A psychiatrist is a doctor who specializes in treating psychiatric conditions such as depression, schizophrenia, bipolar disease, and other conditions that are associated with psychological impairment as a result of brain dysfunction. Some psychiatrists work with other pain medicine physicians, either to help treat the depression and anxiety that so often accompanies chronic pain, or to assist in managing the patient with medication and psychotherapy.

Radiologist

A radiologist is a physician who specializes in administering and interpreting imaging studies of the brain and body, such as radiographs, magnetic resonance imaging (MRI) studies, and computerized tomographic (CT) studies (see Chapter 4). Radiologists provide valuable information to other physicians by helping to elucidate a possible anatomic cause of pain. Some radiologists specialize in administering the therapeutic injections commonly performed in pain management (see Chapter 6).

Rheumatologist

A rheumatologist is a physician who has received specialty training in diagnosing and managing rheumatologic conditions. Rheumatologic conditions generally include disorders of the immune system, such as lupus or rheumatoid arthritis, or degenerative bone conditions such as osteoarthritis of the hips and knees. Some rheumatologists have a special interest in treating low back pain and other spinal conditions. Sacroiliitis, which is discussed in detail in Chapter 14, is an inflammation of part of the lower back that is managed by rheumatologists.

MULTISPECIALTY PAIN CENTER

Multispecialty pain centers are comprised of physicians and other clinicians who specialize in diagnosing and managing patients with chronic pain. Such centers may include pain anesthesiologists, pain neurologists, physiatrists, physical therapists, psychologists, and other practitioners who manage chronic pain. Multispecialty pain centers are generally utilized for patients who suffer with chronic pain, including chronic low back pain.

NONPHYSICIAN CLINICIANS

Nurse

A nurse is a clinician who is trained in the practice of nursing. Nursing is the art and science of providing medical care that is essential to the promotion, maintenance, and restoration of health and well-being in patients. Nursing care also involves the prevention of illness. Nurses work side by side with physicians and often serve as the primary point of contact with the patient. Nurses often develop a specialty, for example pediatric nursing or geriatric nursing. In addition, some nurses receive additional training that qualifies them as a nurse practitioner. Nurse practitioners often work in a physician's office and manage many aspects of a patient's medical care, including the writing of prescription medication.

Physical Therapist

A physical therapist specializes in rehabilitation, but is not a physician. Physical therapists must receive a referral from a physician before treating a patient. Many physical therapists work in their own physical therapy office or practice, and other physical therapists work specifically with a physician. Many physical therapists specialize in sports and orthopedic rehabilitation, and this includes treatment of shoulder, knee, and other joint injuries. Some physical therapists have more specialized training in the spine, but this is not universally so. Some physical therapy techniques center on a concept known as "spine stabilization," which is a progressive therapy that is developed to ensure maximum strength, movement, flexibility, and stability of the spine. In addition, physical therapists specialize in performing various manual techniques that help to ensure proper patient flexibility and muscle balance. Some physical therapists receive training in spinal manipulation.

Physician Assistant

Physician assistants practice medicine under the supervision of physicians and surgeons. Physician assistants are trained to provide diagnostic, therapeutic, and preventive health care services, as delegated by a physician. They take medical histories, examine and treat patients, order and interpret laboratory tests and radiographs, and make diagnoses. They may also treat minor injuries. Under special circumstances, physician assistants may be the principal care providers or even make house calls, after which they must confer with a physician.

Psychologist

A psychologist specializes in psychological counseling. Psychologists are licensed professionals. Some psychologists have a doctorate degree, and others have either a master's degree or a degree as a clinical social worker. Some psychologists specialize in psychoanalysis, and others specialize in cognitive or behavioral therapy. Most pain centers incorporate psychological counseling into their day-to-day practice. For patients who suffer with chronic low back pain, working with a psychologist may be an integral component of proper pain management. Psychologists may help the patient to cope, to learn various behavioral strategies, and to help manage the depression and anxiety that so often accompany chronic pain.

COMPLEMENTARY AND ALTERNATIVE MEDICINE

Practitioners of complementary and alternative medicine (CAM) provide medical care that is, generally speaking, not part of the core curriculum of medical schools. Increasingly, CAM is being incorporated into more traditional medical care and, in such cases, it is more appropriate to utilize the term *integrative medicine*. From one point of view, it might best be said that no such thing as "alternative" medicine exists. There should only be good medicine, and all good medicine should be able to withstand the rigors of the scientific method and evidence-based analysis. Thus, if certain treatment claims are to be made, then such claims should be able to withstand scientific scrutiny so that the treatment results can be reproduced by others.

Acupuncturist

An acupuncturist is a clinician who specializes in acupuncture. Acupuncture has been practiced for more than 4,000 years, beginning as a Chinese medical system. One can become certified in acupuncture in many ways. Some physicians choose to take a specialty course in acupuncture. Others study Traditional Chinese Medicine and still others undertake acupuncture study as part of a broad CAM approach. An acupuncturist uses needles that are inserted into areas of the body lacking a balanced flow of *chi* or life energy force. In addition, acupuncturists may perform a spinning technique with the needle to obtain a relaxation response in a muscle group. Acupuncture is recognized by the World Health Organization (WHO) as a legitimate treatment for certain medical conditions, and many studies have documented the utility of acupuncture in the treatment of low back pain.

Biofeedback Specialist

Biofeedback is a technique that utilizes sensors that are attached to a patient's skin or muscle and then provide signals to a computer. The patient views these signals and is taught how to change them. To change the signals, the patient learns how to relax the skin or muscles. Thus, the computer feedback enables the patient to participate in a relaxation response. Biofeedback specialists are often psychologists who utilize this treatment as one of many ways to help patients obtain a relaxation response.

Chiropractor

A chiropractor is a clinician who has successfully completed chiropractic college. Chiropractors are not medical doctors. They have the initials D.C. (Doctor of Chiropractic) after their names. Chiropractors specialize in spinal manipulation, and the chiropractic approach is spine-centered. Chiropractors view the health of the human being as intimately related to the health of the spine, and this includes the structure and form of the spine. Chiropractors may be the first line of management for patients who suffer with uncomplicated low back pain. Chiropractors should refer to a medical physician specialist when low back pain is not improving with treatment, or if other medical concerns arise. For uncomplicated low back pain, some studies have demonstrated increased satisfaction in those patients who have used chiropractors, when compared with patients who have used family medicine physicians, internists, or orthopedic surgeons as part of their initial low back care.

Massage Therapist

A massage therapist is a clinician who provides massage therapy. Massage therapists have specialty training in working with various muscle groups, using specific hands-on techniques. Some massage therapists work primarily with the acupuncture meridian points (AMMA therapy). Some massage therapists are more sports-oriented, and others utilize more intuitive techniques such as craniosacral technique and myofascial release. Massage therapy generally is used in conjunction with other treatment modalities for patients who suffer with low back pain.

Reflexologist

A reflexologist is a clinician who specializes in reflexology. Reflexology clinicians have training in applying pressure to certain areas of the body, generally the feet, which are thought to have meridian connections with other areas of the body such as the low back. By applying pressure, the body becomes more relaxed, and *chi* energy becomes more balanced.

SUMMARY POINTS

- Many different types of physicians and other health care providers specialize in managing low back pain. Unfortunately for the patient, no simplistic, universal approach exists for treating this condition.
- For simple low back disorders, many physicians and chiropractors are acceptable for first-line management.
- Both orthopedic surgeons and neurosurgeons who have received specialty training in spine surgery may perform surgery of the lumbar spine.
- Patients who have chronic pain should seek help from a pain medicine specialist or from a pain center.
- Complementary and alternative medicine may be incorporated into good medical practice within an integrative approach.

CHAPTER 4

Imaging and Diagnostic Studies

For patients who present with uncomplicated low back pain, a clinician may begin treatment without obtaining a diagnostic study. However, for more severe low back pain, for low back pain that has persisted beyond a few weeks, or for low back pain with other associated symptoms such as fever, chills, weight loss, or a neurologic abnormality, imaging and diagnostic studies become necessary. In today's world of managed care, physicians often must follow certain protocols before obtaining an imaging and diagnostic study, especially for uncomplicated low back pain. Such a protocol often includes verifying that a patient has undergone physical therapy for at least 4 weeks and has not improved with such therapy, thereby justifying the need for further evaluation.

RADIOGRAPHS

A plain radiograph (x-ray film) is usually the first imaging study of a patient who complains of low back pain. Radiographs provide essential but limited information. A radiograph is obtained by a machine emitting radioactive energy. This energy penetrates the patient's body and interacts with a plate placed behind the patient's body (Figure 4.1). A radiographic picture can provide useful information about the general health of a bone, whether a bone has developed a fracture, the alignment of the spine, and degenerative changes of the bone or spine.

Radiographs do not provide reliable information about lumbar discs, nerve roots, or spinal musculature. Some clinicians tell patients that they have looked at the radiographic picture and have diagnosed a pinched nerve, but a radiograph can only provide information about the bone itself. Each time a patient receives a radiograph, he is exposed to radiation energy, and the amount of radiation energy exposure is greater for a

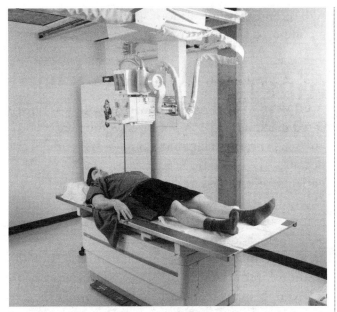

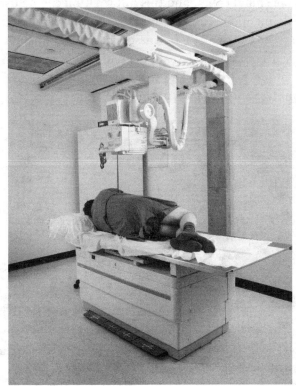

FIGURE 4.1
*A patient undergoing
a radiograph.*

radiograph than for a more specialized test such as a computed tomography (CT) scan.

COMPUTED TOMOGRAPHY SCAN

A CT scan utilizes radiation energy with a sophisticated machine and computerized equipment to provide a three-dimensional image (Figure 4.2). Because the radiation energy is finely focused, patients receive less radiation energy than from a plain radiograph. CT scans can provide good information about the health of a bone, as can a radiograph. In addition, CT scans provide reasonably good information about the lumbar disc and the relationship of the disc and bone to the nerve root. CT scans provide reliable information about the size of the spinal canal, and this information can be used to define more completely any diseases of the bone. CT scans provide a fair assessment of spinal muscles. To obtain a CT scan, the patient lies in a supine or prone position. The test usually takes 15 to 20 minutes, and the patient must lie still.

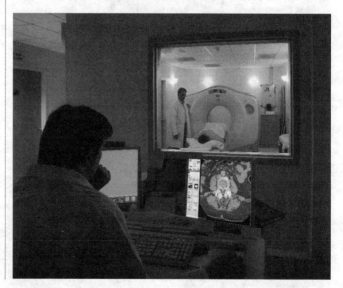

FIGURE 4.2
A view from the computerized terminal room of a patient undergoing a CT scan.

CT scans are not interchangeable with magnetic resonance imaging (MRI), which is discussed next. CT scans provide superior imaging information regarding subtle spinal fractures when compared to MRI. CT scans become necessary as an imaging study when patients have a pacemaker or other mechanical device, because the MRI can cause device malfunction. MRI studies provide superior information about the spinal canal, nerve roots, lumbar discs, and the spinal musculature when compared to CT scans.

MAGNETIC RESONANCE IMAGING

Magnetic resonance imaging (MRI) has revolutionized health care. MRI studies utilize magnetic energy, which is delivered in various sequences, while the patient is lying, sitting, or standing in an appropriate MRI machine. The MRI machine is connected to sophisticated computerized terminals, which interpret the manner in which the magnetic energy interacts with the body, thus producing an image. Some MRI machines are closed, which means that the patient is placed in a rather confined space. Other MRI machines are open, and the space is much less confined, although the image quality and resolution are somewhat diminished (Figure 4.3).

MRI studies provide excellent information regarding the health of the lumbar disc, the nerves, the spinal canal, the spinal musculature, and diseases of the spine. MRI studies usually are performed in patients who have complicated low back presentations, or in patients with ongoing low back or sciatica pain that has not responded successfully to physical therapy or a similar management.

Previously, patients undergoing spinal surgery needed to undergo a *myelogram*, but MRI studies often suffice as the definitive imaging study prior to anticipated spinal surgery. Patients with a pacemaker or similar implantable medical device cannot undergo an MRI study, because the magnetic field can cause the device to malfunction.

MYELOGRAM

A myelogram is a study in which a trained radiologist places a radio-opaque dye into the spinal canal. This is usually performed by way of a lumbar puncture although, under special circumstances, a cervical punc-

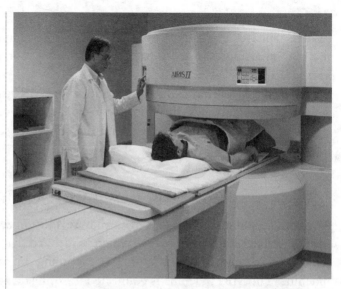

FIGURE 4.3
A patient undergoing an open MRI scan.

ture may be performed. Once the dye is inserted into the spinal canal, a specialized radiograph machine is used, and serial pictures provide an image of the dye in relationship to the nerve roots and the lumbar discs (Figure 4.4).

Generally, a myelogram is followed by a CT scan and, because the dye is in the spinal canal, a post-

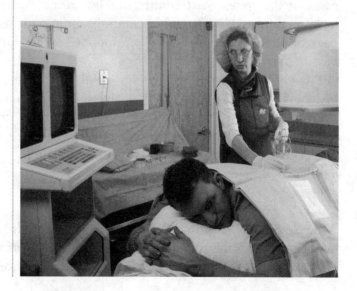

FIGURE 4.4
A patient undergoing a myelogram.

myelogram CT scan provides superior information about the relationship of the spinal joint to the nerve roots than does a plain CT scan. Myelograms are utilized when a diagnosis is in question, for example in the case of a possible spinal tumor or a neurologic condition of the spine that has not been adequately assessed by way of other imaging studies. Some spinal surgeons insist on a myelogram as a definitive test before surgery, but for the most part, MRI has replaced the myelogram in this regard.

DISCOGRAM

A discogram is a procedure in which a radiologist or pain medicine specialist trained in this procedure inserts dye into the lumbar disc. Upon injecting dye into the disc, the pressure within the disc suddenly increases. If the patient's back pain is caused from a faulty disc, then the sudden increase in pressure will reproduce the pain. This is known as *concordant pain*, which means that the patient's pain symptoms are reproduced by the procedure. After dye is inserted into the disc, a plain radiograph and a CT scan are performed, and this allows a detailed analysis of the anatomy of the disc.

Discograms are sometimes performed prior to performing surgery for lumbar degenerative disc disease (see Chapter 11). The surgeon may want to confirm that the degenerative disc is responsible for pain, and he may also want to study other discs to help decide upon the extent of surgery to be performed. It is important to note that a discogram does not replace good clinical judgment, but rather helps to confirm what is already suspected by the physician.

ULTRASOUND

Ultrasound is a technique in which sound waves are delivered through a probe. The manner in which the sound waves interact with the soft tissues results in an image that is interpreted by a clinician. Ultrasound is used much more often in Europe than in the United States for muscular and spinal conditions. In the United States, clinicians generally rely more on MRI studies. An ultrasound can provide very useful information about the state of a muscle, including whether the muscle has an associated tear or tendonitis.

BONE SCAN

A bone scan is performed following the injection of a radioactive substance into the vein. The patient then lies under a machine that produces an image based on the interaction of the injected substance with the bones. Bone scans are extremely effective as a screening tool for patients with suspected bone cancer or bone infection. When patients have low back pain of unclear cause, a bone scan may be ordered to rule out a serious medical cause of low back pain.

A single-photon emission computed tomography (SPECT) bone scan is a more specialized, regional study. This scan is used to judge if subtle abnormalities are present in a specified area of the body, such as the spinal joint. For patients who have undergone lumbar fusion, but who have ongoing, mechanical low back pain, a SPECT bone scan may provide evidence of hardware loosening, meaning that the fusion is not solid.

ELECTROMYOGRAPHY AND NERVE CONDUCTION STUDIES

Nerve conduction studies are based on the premise that a peripheral nerve can be stimulated by a device placed over the skin. The response of the nerve can then be measured by electrodes (similar to electrocardiogram electrodes) placed strategically along the path of the nerve. The velocity and amplitude of the nerve response is measured and interpreted.

Electromyography (EMG) studies are performed by inserting a needle under the skin, and the muscle response to the needle is viewed on a specialized computer screen (Figure 4.5). The physician interprets this response and can discern whether the muscle is responding normally or abnormally. Abnormal responses must be interpreted further; they may be the result of an injury to the nerve or an underlying neurologic disease.

EMG and nerve conduction studies are usually performed as part of the same test because the information obtained is complementary. EMG and nerve conduction studies should be performed by physicians who have received specialty training in such tests (neurologists and some physiatrists). Some chiropractors and other health care practitioners perform these tests without specialty training, and they use machines that are not standardized and approved by governing bodies such as the American

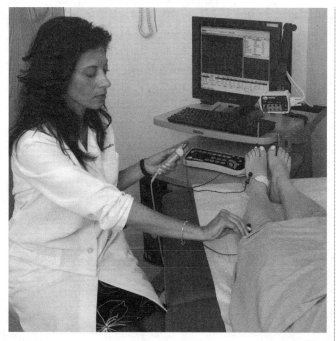

FIGURE 4.5
A patient undergoing EMG and nerve conduction studies.

Academy of Neurology, so the test results can be either meaningless or misleading.

EMG and nerve conduction studies are used diagnostically when a patient with low back pain has suspected nerve damage or muscle damage in conjunction with the low back condition.

SUMMARY POINTS

- Imaging and diagnostic studies aid physicians and other clinicians in managing patients with low back pain.
- Any patient with complicated low back pain must undergo an imaging or diagnostic study.
- Plain radiographs provide basic information about the bones, but provide no details about the nerves or the discs.
- MRI studies provide superior information about the low back anatomy, as well as the nerves,

spinal canal, and the lumbar discs. CT scans provide good detail, and they are sometimes used when assessing for subtle spine fractures or when a patient has a pacemaker.

■ EMG and nerve conduction studies should be performed by physicians who have undergone specialty training in performing these tests.

CHAPTER 5

Medications

A wide variety of medications are utilized in treating patients who suffer with low back pain or related conditions. This chapter includes a summary of commonly used medications, which are grouped according to their general mechanism of action.

FOOD AND DRUG ADMINISTRATION APPROVAL

A discrepancy often exists between the manner in which medications are prescribed by physicians and the strict guidelines outlined by the Food and Drug Administration (FDA). By the time a new medication is approved for marketing to physicians and to the general public, it has been analyzed in numerous studies that are meant to evaluate safety and efficacy. A pharmaceutical company typically applies for approval of a medication for a specific indication. Some typical indications include: for relief of signs and symptoms of osteoarthritis; for the management of acute pain in adults; for the treatment of generalized tonic-clonic seizures; for the treatment of major depressive disorders in adults; and for management of neuropathic pain associated with diabetic peripheral neuropathy.

Even though pharmaceutical companies may market a medication only for its approved indication, physicians may prescribe a medication for nonapproved indications. For example, gabapentin (Neurontin) is an anticonvulsant medication that originally was approved by the FDA for use in a particular type of seizure disorder. Soon after its market availability, physicians began to prescribe gabapentin for other, non-FDA approved uses. One such use is neuropathic pain. There exists a large body of literature supporting the clinical benefit of anticonvulsants in alleviating symptoms of neuropathic pain. Because gabapentin is extremely effective for this use, it became common practice for pain medicine physicians to prescribe gabapentin for neuropathic pain, despite the fact that it was not formally approved for such use. This practice is known as using a medication *off-label*.

In the case of gabapentin, even though numerous physicians were prescribing this medication for pain management, the pharmaceutical company that produced this drug was not allowed to market gabapentin for its use in pain, either to physicians directly or to the general public. The pharmaceutical company later received approval to market this drug for a particular type of neuropathic pain: postherpetic neuralgia, which is neuropathic pain that develops following shingles (a type of herpes infection).

It is important for patients to understand that it is extremely common for physicians to prescribe medications in an off-label manner in pain management. This is more often the case for chronic, neuropathic pain, because few medications have FDA approval for this condition. In this case, it is commonplace to prescribe anticonvulsant and antidepressant medication, for reasons discussed later. Even for acute pain, physicians often prescribe an anti-inflammatory medication in an off-label manner, because most of these drugs only have approval as a treatment for rheumatoid arthritis or osteoarthritis.

NONSTEROIDAL ANTI-INFLAMMATORY DRUGS

How They Work

Nonsteroidal anti-inflammatory drugs (NSAIDs) have pain-relieving, anti-inflammatory, and antipyretic (anti-fever) properties. Although a large number of NSAIDs exist, and although they have a diverse chemical profile, all these medications work in a similar manner. In essence, NSAIDs inhibit what is known as the COX enzyme system. When injury occurs, certain substances are produced by the injured cell. A series of chemical reactions occur, and each reaction depends on an enzyme for its completion. The COX enzyme system is very important in producing compounds known as *prostaglandins*, which are responsible for many of the inflammation, pain, and fever effects following tissue injury. When a medication inhibits the COX system, then the compounds that produce inflammation, pain, and fever following tissue injury are not produced in normal amounts.

The COX system is divided into COX-1 and COX-2, and this division has become the basis for a new class of NSAIDs known as COX-2 inhibitors. The COX-1 system, when inhibited, produces two potentially unwanted side effects:

- COX-1 inhibition prevents *platelets* from functioning normally. Platelets are the first blood products to arrive following any tissue injury that may cause bleeding. Platelets clump around the injury as the first line of defense. If platelets are inhibited, bleeding is more likely to be prolonged.
- COX-1 inhibition inhibits a protective effect on the stomach; therefore, NSAIDs that inhibit COX-1 are more likely to cause stomach irritation, including a bleeding ulcer.

Prior to the introduction of the COX-2–specific NSAIDs, all NSAID medications inhibited both COX-1 and COX-2 enzymes. The specific COX-2 inhibitors entered the American and European market with widespread fanfare because of their ability to relieve inflammation, pain, and fever without the unwanted blood and stomach side effects. However, recent evidence has demonstrated that two of these medications may produce a new side effect of NSAIDs: heart attack and stroke. Because of these potential complications, two of the COX-2 inhibitors have been removed from the market (rofecoxib [Vioxx] and valdecoxib [Bextra]). A third COX-2 inhibitor, celecoxib (Celebrex), does not demonstrate any evidence of an increase in risk of heart attack or stroke, and this medication is considered safe when used in the manner for which it is intended.

Side Effects

Side effects of NSAIDs depend on whether the medication inhibits the COX-1 enzyme. Other than celecoxib (Celebrex), all NSAIDs currently available on the market inhibit the COX-1 enzyme. Inhibition of this enzyme increases the risk of developing stomach irritation, including an ulcer. Stomach irritation is the major limiting side effect of these medications. A bleeding ulcer is a medical emergency, and is potentially life threatening.

Platelet inhibition and enhanced bleeding following injury is usually not a limiting side effect of NSAIDs, but in some cases this is problematic. Patients undergoing surgery or dental work will bleed more if they have recently ingested an NSAID. Epidural injections and other similar pain injections (described in Chapter 6) may not be performed when these medications are inside the body. Patients who take warfarin (Coumadin), a powerful anticoagulant medication, may not take NSAIDs. Aspirin in particular causes a prolonged inhibition of platelets (7 to 10 days), whereas other NSAIDs inhibit platelets for a matter of hours to days, depending on the drug.

Both COX-1 and COX-2 inhibition may slow bone healing. Some studies have shown that bone fractures heal more slowly in patients who ingest NSAIDs. For this reason, spinal surgeons do not prescribe these medications following spinal fusion surgery, because this may delay or prevent proper bone fusion.

Patients who take these medications long-term must undergo kidney and liver function monitoring. NSAID use has been implicated in kidney damage, especially when patients ingest larger than normal doses. In most cases, kidney and liver damage is reversible when these medications are discontinued. In addition to kidney and liver damage, blood pressure may become elevated, and patients may develop swelling in their legs; both of these complications are a reason to discontinue the NSAID medication.

Celecoxib (Celebrex) is unique in that it does not inhibit platelet function, so this medication can be more safely utilized around the time of surgical procedures. Celecoxib causes less stomach irritation than does a traditional NSAID, and it may be protective against colon cancer as well.

Indications in Pain Management

Although most NSAIDs are not FDA-approved for management of acute pain, it is common to utilize these medications for such use. These medications are useful for patients who develop a first attack of low back pain, or for patients who have more chronic low back pain but develop a superimposed attack of more severe pain. NSAIDs also may be used shortly before an activity, such as prolonged standing, that is likely to aggravate a low back condition.

A rational strategy for NSAID use is to take these medications as prescribed for several days to a few weeks following an acute or recurrent bout of low back pain or a related condition. Chronic use of these medications may be ineffective and requires careful monitoring by the prescribing physician. There are times when NSAIDs are prescribed routinely on a long-term basis for patients with chronic low back pain; such use should be discouraged unless compelling evidence shows that long-term use leads to meaningful pain reduction.

The choice of medication is primarily guided by physician comfort. Many physicians become comfortable using certain brand names, so they prefer to start with such medications. Another important consideration is side effect profile, and this consideration is the major determinant in the use of a traditional NSAID versus celecoxib (Celebrex). Other than celecoxib, the benefit and side effect profile are rather similar for the various NSAIDs. For reasons that are not completely understood scientifically, some patients respond much more favorably to a particular NSAID and thus, it does make sense to try a different NSAID when symptoms of pain are not relieved.

COMMONLY PRESCRIBED NONSTEROIDAL ANTI-INFLAMMATORY DRUGS

Table 5.1 lists the most commonly prescribed NSAIDs used in treating low back pain.

Aspirin (Acetylsalicylic Acid, Bayer, Bufferin, Ecotrin, Excedrin)

Aspirin is widely available as an *over-the-counter medication*, which means medication that may be purchased without a physician prescription. Generally speaking, aspirin is tolerated less well than other NSAIDs. Aspirin inhibits platelet function irreversibly, which means that the platelet will not function for its lifespan of approximately 7 to 10 days. Aspirin causes more stomach irritation than do most other NSAIDs, and it must be taken every 4 hours in order to obtain a therapeutic effect of pain and inflammation relief. The therapeutic dose of aspirin for acute low back pain is 650 mg to 1,000 mg every 4 to 6 hours.

TABLE 5.1
Commonly Prescribed Nonsteroidal Anti-Inflammatory Drugs for Low Back Pain

GENERIC NAME	BRAND NAME	STARTING DOSE	MAINTENANCE DOSE
Acetylsalicylic Acid, Aspirin	Bayer, Bufferin, Ecotrin, Excedrin	650-1000mg every 4-6 hours	650-1000mg every 4-6 hours
Celecoxib	Celebrex	400mg	200mg twice daily
Diclofenac	Voltaren, Voltaren XR	100-150mg	100-150mg daily, in 1-2 doses
Diflunisal	Dolobid	1000mg	250-500mg twice daily
Etodolac	Lodine XL	400mg 3 times daily	200-400mg 2-3 times daily
Ibuprofen	Advil, Motrin, Nuprin	200-800mg 3-4 times daily	200-800mg 3-4 times daily
Indomethacin	Indocin	25mg 2-3 times daily	25-75mg 2-3 times daily
Ketorolac	Toradol	Intramuscular: 60mg Intravenous: 30mg Oral: 10mg 2-3 times daily	10mg 2-3 times daily, short-term
Meloxicam	Mobic	15mg	7.5-15mg daily, in 1-2 doses
Nabumetone	Relafen	1000mg	500-1000mg twice daily
Naproxen, Naproxen Sodium	Aleve, Anaprox, Naprosyn	250-1000mg	250-500mg twice daily

Celecoxib (Celebrex)

Celecoxib has withstood intense scrutiny as a COX-2 inhibitor drug, and all data to date indicate that this medication is safe when taken as recommended. Celecoxib does not inhibit platelet function, which is an advantage for patients who may be undergoing surgery or who are taking other blood-thinning medications. Celecoxib is well-tolerated and causes less stomach irritation than traditional NSAIDs. Celecoxib is indicated for acute pain in adults. This means that celecoxib is approved not only for medical conditions such as rheumatoid arthritis and osteoarthritis, but also for sudden pain that may be related to a muscle spasm or other back problems. The recommended initial dose is 400 mg, followed by 200 mg every 12 hours for several days to weeks.

Diclofenac (Voltaren, Voltaren-XR)

Diclofenac passes through the liver before it is effective as an NSAID and, for this reason, a higher incidence of liver injury occurs with this medication. Diclofenac may be taken up to four times daily for the first day of use. Thereafter, it is prescribed as a once- or twice-daily medication. Usual starting dose is 100 to 150 mg, followed by 100 to 150 mg daily in 1–2 doses.

Diflunisal (Dolobid)

Diflunisal is chemically similar to aspirin, but may be slightly better tolerated in the stomach than is aspirin. The usual starting dose is 1,000 mg, followed by 250 to 500 mg twice daily.

Etodolac (Lodine XL)

Etodolac is more highly specific to COX-2 than it is to COX-1 and, for this reason, fewer stomach side effects may occur. Etodolac will, however, inhibit platelet function. The usual starting dose is 400 mg three times daily, followed by 200 to 400 mg two to three times daily.

Ibuprofen (Advil, Motrin, Nuprin)

Like aspirin, ibuprofen is an over-the-counter medication, meaning that it can be purchased without a physician's prescription. Larger-dose formulations (400 to 800 mg) are prescribed by a physician. Ibuprofen commonly is used for acute pain, and it must be taken three to four times daily. Sometimes, a single dose is used to prevent pain; for example, some patients utilize a single dose before performing an activity (such as prolonged standing) that might provoke pain. Side effects are similar to other NSAIDs, but are less common at lower doses. The usual starting dose depends on the severity of pain and can range from 200 mg three to four times daily for mild pain, to 800 mg three to four times daily for more severe pain. The longer-term dose ranges from 200 mg to 800 mg three to four times daily.

Indomethacin (Indocin)

Indomethacin is used less commonly for acute low back pain, and is utilized more specifically for gout (a painful inflammation of joints, especially the great toe) or for some severe headache conditions. Indomethacin has a relatively high incidence of stomach and kidney side effects. The usual starting dose is 25 mg two to three times daily, with a similar maintenance dose that may be increased, as tolerated and as needed, under strict physician supervision.

Ketorolac (Toradol)

Ketorolac is unique because it is currently the only NSAID in the United States that may be given as an intravenous or intramuscular injection. For severe, acute pain, an injection of ketorolac may be highly effective, and this is often a strategy employed by emergency-room physicians. The oral form of ketorolac is less effective for controlling pain and, because of a relatively high incidence of side effects, its long-term use is limited and is not recommended.

Meloxicam (Mobic)

This medication is sometimes inaccurately described as a "relative" COX-2 inhibitor. However, in normal therapeutic doses, meloxicam inhibits COX-1, similarly to other NSAIDs, with similar stomach and platelet side effects. Usual starting dose is 15 mg, followed by 7.5 mg to 15 mg per day, given in one or two doses.

Nabumetone (Relafen)

Like etodolac, nabumetone is more specific to COX-2 than it is to COX-1 and, for this reason, some studies have demonstrated that nabumetone is less likely to cause stomach irritation. However, nabumetone does have an effect on platelet inhibition, so some COX-1 activity is present. The usual starting dose is 1,000 mg, followed by 500 mg to 1,000 mg twice daily.

Naproxen and Naproxen Sodium
(Aleve, Anaprox, Naprosyn)

Like ibuprofen, naproxen preparations are available over-the-counter or, in larger doses, as a prescription medication. The usual starting dose is

250 mg for mild pain, and 1,000 mg for more severe pain. A maintenance dose is 250 mg to 500 mg twice daily.

THE SPECIAL CASE OF ACETAMINOPHEN (TYLENOL)

Acetaminophen is not a NSAID. Although acetaminophen has pain-relieving and fever-reducing properties similar to other NSAIDs, it has no effect on inflammation. Acetaminophen has no significant stomach toxicity, and no effect on platelet function. Acetaminophen is an often underutilized alternative to NSAID use. The usual dosage is 350 mg to 1,000 mg, and it must be taken three to four times daily. Liver damage is a major concern with acetaminophen use. An acute overdose may cause liver failure and death. Long-term use in doses greater than 2,000 mg to 3,000 mg per day requires physician monitoring of liver function.

MUSCLE RELAXANTS

How They Work

Muscle relaxants commonly are prescribed for patients who develop acute low back pain, especially with associated muscle spasm. Muscle relaxants work by inhibiting the brain or spinal cord mechanisms that enhance muscle tone, and they lead to a relaxed state in the muscle. Some muscle relaxants are effective in reducing spasticity, which is a condition that develops in certain neurologic diseases such as multiple sclerosis, cerebral palsy, and spinal cord injury. *Spasticity* means that the muscle tone is quite stiff, and finely controlled muscle movements are limited. Most muscle relaxants effectively reduce muscle spasms but have no effect on spasticity. Muscle relaxants are utilized to treat acute and chronic low back conditions.

Side Effects

Most muscle relaxants are well tolerated from the point of view of the stomach and gastrointestinal track. They do not affect bleeding time. Although a low incidence of kidney or liver damage occurs, patients taking these medications long-term should be monitored through blood tests of liver and kidney function. The most common side effects, which limit their use, are dizziness, mental clouding, confusion, and fatigue. These side effects vary from medication to medication, which means that some patients may tolerate one type of muscle relaxant more than they do another.

Indications in Pain Management

Patients who develop acute pain often have associated muscle spasm. Regardless of the cause of acute pain, reducing muscle spasm helps to reduce pain. In addition, reducing muscle spasm prevents unwanted pressure on the spine, because muscle spasm can affect the proper function of the spinal joint and lumbar discs.

Some patients have chronic muscle spasm, usually in association with a chronic, neuropathic pain condition. Normally, following an acute injury, muscle spasm lasts for days to weeks, then resolves. Chronic muscle spasm indicates that the patient's physiology has changed, consistent with a neuropathic pain condition. Muscle relaxants should not be used as a stand-alone treatment for muscle spasm in patients with chronic pain, but rather should be part of a more comprehensive treatment plan, including physical therapy, exercise, and mindfulness.

COMMONLY PRESCRIBED MUSCLE RELAXANTS

Table 5.2 lists those muscle relaxants commonly prescribed in the treatment of low back pain.

Baclofen (Lioresal)

Baclofen is similar to the brain chemical gamma aminobutyric acid (GABA). GABA pathways are very involved in controlling muscle tone and spasticity. Baclofen is an effective antispasticity medication, although it usually is not a first-line medication for acute muscle spasm. Baclofen often is used long-term to treat patients with spasticity and, in some cases, it is used in neuropathic pain conditions. Baclofen is unique in that it can be delivered as an infusion directly into the spinal canal via a pump (intrathecal delivery), similar to a morphine pump. For patients with severe spasticity, or for patients with severe neuropathic pain and muscle spasm, baclofen may be a highly effective intrathecal

TABLE 5.2
Commonly Prescribed Muscle Relaxants for Low Back Pain

GENERIC NAME	BRAND NAME	STARTING DOSE	MAINTENANCE DOSE
Baclofen	Lioresal	5-10mg	5-20mg, 3-4 times daily
Carisoprodol	Soma, Soma Compound, Soma Compound with Codeine	350mg	350mg 3-4 times daily
Chlorzoxazone	Paraflex, Parafon Forte	250-500mg	250-500mg 3-4 times daily
Cyclobenzaprine	Flexeril	10mg	10mg 3-4 times daily
Diazepam	Valium	2-5mg	2-5mg 3-4 times daily
Metaxalone	Skelaxin	400-800mg	400-800mg 3-4 times daily
Methocarbamol	Robaxin, Robaxisal	500-750mg	500-750mg 3-4 times daily
Orphenadrine	Norflex, Norgesic Norgesic Forte	100mg	100mg twice daily
Tizanidine	Zanaflex	2-4 mg	4-36mg in 3-4 divided doses

medication. The normal oral dose is 5 mg to 20 mg three to four times daily. The most common side effects are drowsiness, dizziness, confusion, and disequilibrium. If baclofen is stopped abruptly, patients may develop hallucinations.

Carisoprodol (Soma, Soma Compound, Soma Compound with Codeine)

Carisoprodol inhibits pathways in the spinal cord that cause muscle spasm, and it has some sedating effects as well. Carisoprodol does not have an effect on spasticity. Carisoprodol is an effective medication for acute muscle spasm, and is utilized for some patients with chronic pain. Carisoprodol may be utilized alone (Soma), or in combination with aspirin (Soma Compound) or aspirin and codeine (Soma Compound with Codeine). The normal dose is 350 mg three to four times daily. The most common side effects are drowsiness, dizziness, and mental clouding.

Chlorzoxazone (Paraflex, Parafon Forte)

Chlorzoxazone inhibits pathways in the brain and spinal cord, which leads to muscle relaxation. Chlorzoxazone is indicated for acute muscle spasm, and does not reduce muscle spasticity. The normal dose is 250 mg to 500 mg three to four times daily. The most common side effects are dizziness and drowsiness.

Cyclobenzaprine (Flexeril)

Cyclobenzaprine is related chemically to the tricyclic antidepressant medications, which are discussed in later sections. Cyclobenzaprine inhibits the brain pathways that cause muscle spasm, but does not affect spasticity. Because of its similarity to the tricyclic antidepressant medications, cyclobenzaprine may have some pain-relieving effects in addition to reducing local muscle spasm. (The pain-relieving effects of antidepressants are discussed later in this chapter.) Cyclobenzaprine is an effective medication for acute muscle spasm, and it is utilized for some patients with chronic pain. The normal dose is 10 mg three to four times daily. The most common side effects are drowsiness, dizziness, and a dry mouth. Some patients may develop urinary retention, so this medication should be used cautiously in male patients with an enlarged prostate.

Diazepam (Valium)

Diazepam is a unique muscle relaxant, because it is also a powerful sedative and antianxiety medication. Diazepam also is used to treat seizures. Diazepam reduces both muscle spasm and spasticity, and it is sometimes used long term to treat patients with brain or spinal cord injury. For patients with acute, severe pain and associated anxiety, diazepam is highly effective in aiding patients to rest while reducing muscle spasm. However, diazepam is a highly addictive medication, so long-term use is reserved for special circumstances such as spasticity, or in some cases of severe neuropathic pain. The normal dose is 2 mg to 5 mg, three to four times daily. In special cases, diazepam also can be administered as an injection into the muscle or directly into the bloodstream as an intravenous infusion. The most common side effects are drowsiness, dizziness, and confusion.

Metaxalone (Skelaxin)

The exact manner by which metaxalone produces its effects is not clear, but it probably works by depressing the brain activity involved in the response to sudden muscle injury. Metaxalone is indicated for sudden painful muscle conditions. Metaxalone does not reduce muscle spasticity. The normal dose is 400 mg to 800 mg three to four times daily, as needed. The most common side effects are dizziness, drowsiness, nausea, and irritability.

Methocarbamol (Robaxin, Robaxisal)

The exact manner by which methocarbamol produces its effects is not clear, but it is likely that methocarbamol works by depressing some brain activity that may be involved in muscle-spasm pathways. Methocarbamol does not reduce spasticity. The normal dose is 500 mg to 750 mg three to four times daily. Methocarbamol may be used alone (Robaxin) or in combination with aspirin (Robaxisal). In special cases and under physician supervision, methocarbamol also may be injected into the muscle or directly into the bloodstream as an intravenous infusion. The most common side effects are drowsiness, dizziness, and nausea.

Orphenadrine
(Norflex, Norgesic, Norgesic Forte)

Orphenadrine has properties somewhat similar to diphenhydramine (Benadryl), which is an antihistamine. Orphenadrine may reduce muscle spasm by depressing the brainstem activity that is involved in responding to acute muscle injury. Orphenadrine also may have some direct pain-relieving effect. Orphenadrine may be used alone (Norflex), or in combination with aspirin (Norgesic) or aspirin and caffeine (Norgesic Forte). The normal dose is 100 mg twice daily. In special circumstances and under the supervision of a physician, orphenadrine may be injected directly into the muscle or into the bloodstream as an intravenous infusion. The most common side effects are drowsiness and dizziness. In addition, patients may experience dry mouth, blurred vision, and urinary retention.

Tizanidine (Zanaflex)

Tizanidine is a powerful muscle relaxant effective in reducing spasticity. Tizanidine binds to receptors in the brain and produces a combination of effects that can lead to reduced muscle spasm, reduced spasticity, and pain relief. Because tizanidine changes some pathways that are involved in chronic pain, it is often utilized long-term to treat patients with neuropathic pain. Tizanidine also is utilized to treat chronic headache. Tizanidine is a more powerful medication than are most muscle relaxants, and it must be started very slowly. The normal starting dose is 2 mg to 4 mg once daily, usually at night. The dose is then increased by 2 mg to 4 mg every 4 to 7 days, taken three to four times daily. The highest target doses range from 24 mg to 36 mg daily. Side effects are common and include dizziness, drowsiness, confusion, dry mouth, nightmares, and hallucinations. Blood pressure should be monitored, because some patients develop hypotension (low blood pressure).

NARCOTIC ANALGESICS

How They Work

Analgesics are medications that provide pain relief. Narcotic analgesics (opioids) are the most potent prescription analgesics. Narcotic analgesics work by binding to the narcotic receptors that are part of the normal makeup of the human body. A *receptor* is part of the body, located on a cell, which responds to a certain type of chemical. When the chemical and receptor interact, a "lock-and-key" type of response occurs, which means that a particular type of chemical will only bind to a matching receptor. When this happens, a specific reaction occurs. When narcotic receptors are activated in our brain and spinal cord, we have less appreciation of and care less about pain, which results in analgesia.

Depending on the strength of the narcotic analgesic and the state of the individual's receptors, the effect can range from mild pain relief to coma. Over time, repeated use of narcotic analgesics leads to a change in the individual's drug tolerance. Thus, the same dose has less of an effect, both with regard to pain relief and to any accompanying side effects. This phenomenon is known as *drug tolerance*.

Side Effects

The biggest side effects of narcotic analgesics are constipation, nausea and vomiting, and mental clouding. Constipation occurs because narcotic (opiate) receptors also are located within the intestines and, when these receptors are activated by narcotic analgesics, the effect is to slow down intestinal motility. Nausea and vomiting may develop acutely because of the activation of certain receptors in the brain. Fortunately, most patients develop tolerance to nausea and vomiting from narcotic analgesics.

With regard to mental clouding, patients who are naïve to narcotics may become confused, may feel lethargic, or may feel spacey after taking these medications. In elderly patients, or in patients with mild dementia, mental clouding may be associated with severe confusion or even delirium. When patients take narcotic analgesics long term, for example for chronic pain, the mental clouding effects usually disappear. Indeed, studies have demonstrated that patients may function normally with regard to mental alertness when they take narcotic analgesics over an extended period. Thus, such patients may be able to drive a motor vehicle without any restrictions.

Indications in Pain Management

Unfortunately, an inherent bias exists against prescribing narcotic analgesics for patients who suffer with pain. Family members, friends, or patients themselves may frown upon the need to take such medications. Physicians may become judgmental against patients who have been prescribed such medications by another doctor, or against patients who request such medications. In addition, the Drug Enforcement Agency (DEA) has begun to investigate physicians who prescribe large quantities of these medications, even when the prescriptions are legitimate. Thus, there exists a general sense of fear with regard to prescribing and taking narcotic analgesics.

Despite the negativity surrounding narcotic analgesics, they are an extremely important part of pain management when treating patients with moderate or severe pain. The fact remains that these medications are the most potent class of pain relievers available. For this reason, narcotic analgesic use should be considered for patients who suffer with moderate or severe pain. Generally, the patient will require such a medication for 1 to 2 weeks. In this instance, a short-acting narcotic analgesic should be used. Short-acting means that the effect of the narcotic lasts no more than 4 to 6 hours.

A place also is reserved for the long-term use of narcotic analgesics in patients with chronic pain. Many years ago, it was felt that the long-term use of narcotic analgesics should be reserved only for patients with debilitating cancer pain. Now, the medical community has embraced the notion that long-term narcotic use also may be appropriate for *nonmalignant pain*, which means pain that is not caused by cancer. In this case, the decision to treat with these medications should be made by a pain medicine specialist, and such medication should be part of a multidisciplinary management plan.

Because pain is subjective in nature, and because there is no way to measure its intensity, the most important indicator to follow in patients who receive narcotic analgesics is functional improvement. For acute pain, this means that patients are suffering less and are better able to move about without suffering. For patients with chronic pain, functional improvement may be defined physically, emotionally, and behaviorally. If narcotic analgesics improve function in patients with chronic pain, it is also important to utilize a long-acting medication, so that pain relief is sustained, and patients are not required to seek medication every few hours. Such long-acting medications can last anywhere from 8 hours to 3 days per dosing, depending on the medication and the patient's individual response.

In addition to the obvious pain-relieving advantage of using a long-acting narcotic analgesic in patients with chronic pain, there is the psychological benefit that patients are not chasing after their pain throughout the day, constantly searching for medication every 3 to 4 hours. Even in patients who achieve relatively good pain control using long-acting narcotic analgesics, *breakthrough pain* may develop from time to time, which means that the patient develops a sudden worsening of pain despite taking a narcotic analgesic. If breakthrough pain develops only periodically, then it is appropriate to treat this pain with a short-acting narcotic analgesic. If breakthrough pain develops regularly, then the dose of the long-acting narcotic analgesic may need to be increased.

It is common and advisable for physicians who prescribe narcotic analgesics for long-term use in patients with nonmalignant pain to ask patients to sign a *narcotic contract*. The essential provisions of a narcotic contract are that the patient will only receive narcotic analgesic medications from one physician (or physician group), will only take the medication in the manner prescribed, will fill prescriptions from the same pharmacy, will follow-up for a physician visit at least monthly, and will be subject to drug screening tests from time to time. Such contracts protect the physician's practice and help to establish important guidelines for the patient.

COMMONLY PRESCRIBED NARCOTIC ANALGESICS

Unlike other medications, no simple "recommended dose" exists for narcotic analgesics. Usually, physicians begin with a low-potency medication, then increase the dose based on the patient's needs. In this section, dosing is discussed in a limited manner, because dosing is so highly variable with this class of drugs.

Fentanyl (Actiq, Duragesic)

Fentanyl is a powerful narcotic analgesic that has unique properties that allow it to be formulated as a transdermal preparation (a skin patch) or transmucosal preparation (as a lollipop). In either case, the medication is not swallowed as a pill. Fentanyl also is used intravenously during anesthesia.

When used as a skin patch, transdermal fentanyl (Duragesic) is absorbed through the skin continuously over a period of 3 days. Before beginning transdermal fentanyl, the physician should have an idea of the underlying narcotic need and tolerance of the patient. Dosing tables allow physicians to calculate the proper amount of a fentanyl skin patch based on the amount of shorter-acting narcotic analgesics the patient is taking. Transdermal fentanyl is ideal for patients with chronic pain, especially those who tolerate oral medications poorly.

As opposed to transdermal fentanyl, transmucosal fentanyl (Actiq) is extremely short acting. The patient sucks on a lollipop-type preparation, and some of the medication is absorbed immediately through the cheek. Some pain relief occurs within 5 to 10 minutes. Transmucosal fentanyl is ideal for patients who develop sudden bouts of severe pain and therefore require pain relief more acutely. Transmucosal fentanyl may be used as the only narcotic analgesic, or as a medication for breakthrough pain in patients who are also using long-acting narcotic analgesics.

Hydrocodone (Lorcet, Lortab, Norco, Vicodin, Vicoprofen)

Hydrocodone is a lower-potency narcotic analgesic that usually is combined with acetaminophen (Lorcet, Lortab, Norco, Vicodin) or ibuprofen (Vicoprofen). Common dosing is 5 mg, 7.5 mg, and 10 mg. Patients with moderate to severe pain who do not respond to other medications often are prescribed hydrocodone. The usual starting dose is 5 mg every 4 hours as needed.

Hydromorphone (Dilaudid)

Hydromorphone is a powerful narcotic analgesic that may be given intravenously or subcutaneously (into the skin) for hospitalized patients who develop severe pain. As an oral preparation, hydromorphone is short-acting, with pain relief lasting 3 to 4 hours. For patients with severe pain, hydromorphone is appropriate short term. Long term, hydromorphone should be used for breakthrough pain only.

Methadone

Methadone is a powerful narcotic analgesic that also binds to a non-narcotic receptor that is important in controlling pain (the NMDA receptor). Methadone was used in a highly successful manner decades ago as a treatment for heroin addicts, and such use continues today. Because methadone is associated culturally with heroin addicts, many patients and physicians are reluctant to utilize this medication.

Pain medicine specialists are beginning to utilize methadone more and more. Not only is methadone a powerful long-acting oral medication (dosed two to three times per day), it is also cheaper than most other narcotic analgesics. Methadone is an ideal drug for patients with chronic pain who have developed tolerance to other narcotic analgesics.

Morphine (Avinza, Kadian, MSIR, MS Contin, Oramorph)

Morphine is the prototypical narcotic analgesic, which means it is the narcotic to which all others are compared. Morphine can be given orally, intravenously, or subcutaneously. As an oral drug, it is formulated as a short-acting liquid (Oramorph) or pill (MSIR), or as a long-acting pill (Avinza, Kadian, and MS Contin). For hospitalized patients, intravenous or subcutaneous morphine is an ideal medication when treating severe pain. Otherwise, oral morphine preparations are prescribed when patients with severe pain have not responded to lower-potency narcotic analgesics. The short-acting preparations last 3 to 4 hours, and the long-acting preparations last 8 to 12 hours.

Oxycodone (Combunox, Endocet, Endodan, OxyContin, Percocet, Percodan, Roxicet)

Oxycodone is a commonly prescribed narcotic analgesic for patients who develop sudden, moderate to severe pain. As a start-up medication, it is commonly prescribed in combination with acetaminophen (Endocet, Percocet, Roxicet), aspirin (Endodan, Percodan), or ibuprofen (Combunox), in 5-mg, 7.5-mg, and 10-mg preparations. These short-acting preparations last 3 to 4 hours. Long-acting oxycodone (OxyContin) provides pain relief for 8 to 12 hours.

Propoxyphene (Darvocet-N 50 or -N 100, Darvon, Darvon N, Darvon Compound-65)

Propoxyphene is a lower-potency narcotic analgesic commonly prescribed for patients with moderate pain. It is prepared alone (Darvon, Darvon N), in combination with acetaminophen (Darvocet-N 50, Darvocet-N 100), or in combination with aspirin and caffeine (Darvon Compound-65). The usual dose is one to two tablets every 3 to 4 hours as needed. Darvon Compound-65 often is used to treat patients who suffer with migraine and other headache conditions.

Tramadol (Ultracet, Ultram, UltramER)

Tramadol is a unique medication in that it binds to an opiate receptor and also acts on two other brain pathways that influence pain. Although tramadol is sometimes classified as a non-narcotic analgesic, for all practical purposes it is a lower-potency narcotic analgesic. It is prepared alone

(Ultram) or in combination with acetaminophen (Ultracet). The usual dose is one to two tablets every 4 to 6 hours. UltramER is a once-daily preparation that is utilized in patients who would otherwise require multiple doses of tramadol on a daily basis. In addition to the usual narcotic side effects, tramadol has been reported to cause seizures in a small proportion of patients.

ANTIDEPRESSANTS

How They Work

Antidepressants have become an important tool in the treatment of patients who suffer with chronic pain. Antidepressant medications are not indicated for the treatment of acute pain. Antidepressant medications are useful for treating patients with chronic pain because they offer some pain-relieving qualities in and of themselves; they also are helpful in treating underlying depression and anxiety, which frequently accompany chronic pain.

Antidepressant medications are classified according to their mechanism of action. The older antidepressant medications are limited by a wide number of side effects. Newer antidepressant medications have fewer side effects because of a more refined mechanism of action.

With regard to pain control, antidepressant medications work by modifying certain brain pathways that influence pain. For example, the *serotonin* and *norepinephrine* pathways have important effects on inhibiting the spinal cord's response to chronic pain signals. Serotonin and norepinephrine are brain chemicals that also are involved in controlling mood. Thus, an antidepressant medication that influences serotonin and norepinephrine can have an effect on mood as well as pain.

It was discovered many years ago that diabetic patients who suffer with severe, burning nerve pain may develop significant pain alleviation after taking a low dose of amitriptyline, which is one of the first antidepressants marketed in the United States. This pain-relieving effect occurred independent of any effect on mood. Indeed, amitriptyline could be utilized in a very low dose, one that was not even effective for controlling mood. Around the same time that this clinical discovery was made, there were many other important scientific discoveries regarding the various brain

pathways. This included an understanding that the body has its own opiate receptors (as discussed earlier, in the section on narcotic analgesics),
and that these opiate receptors interact with serotonin and norepinephrine pathways. It became clear over time that the opiate, serotonin, and
norepinephrine pathways have a profound effect on the individual's perception of pain.

In general, antidepressant medications work by preventing the breakdown of chemicals such as serotonin and norepinephrine. Other brain
chemicals influence mood as well, including dopamine. *Dopamine* is a
neurochemical that is important in experiences of extreme joy, for example religious ecstasy or orgasm. Dopamine is also an important chemical
in mediating the effects of addiction to drugs such as nicotine. Some antidepressants influence the availability of dopamine and produce their
effects in ways similar to antidepressants that influence the availability of
serotonin and norepinephrine.

It is easiest to categorize antidepressants as follows: (a) tricyclic antidepressants; (b) selective serotonin reuptake inhibitors; (c) serotonin–norepinephrine reuptake inhibitors; (d) other antidepressants.

Although antidepressants may help to diminish pain perception, it is
important to understand that the vast majority of patients with chronic
pain also suffer with associated depression and anxiety. It is difficult, if
not impossible, to treat chronic pain effectively if depression and anxiety
persist. Thus, utilizing an antidepressant medication to treat the depression and anxiety that coexist with chronic pain is extremely important.
Such medications also should be coupled with behavioral strategies and
psychological intervention.

Side Effects

Tricyclic Antidepressants

Tricyclic antidepressants were the first group of antidepressants widely
marketed for the treatment of depression and anxiety. They are much less
specific than are the newer-generation antidepressants. In addition to
increasing the availability of serotonin and norepinephrine, they also
influence other brain chemicals, which leads to their considerable side
effects. Tricyclic antidepressants usually cause weight gain. Sedation is

often the most limiting side effect. Patients frequently develop a dry mouth, constipation, blurred vision, and urinary retention. In some cases, patients become confused. Sexual side effects, especially loss of libido (sexual drive), are common. In patients with a history of heart disease, tricyclic antidepressants must be used cautiously because they can sometimes lead to an irregular heartbeat.

Selective Serotonin Reuptake Inhibitors (SSRIs)

Selective serotonin reuptake inhibitors (SSRIs) have revolutionized the treatment of depression because of their considerable specificity, effectiveness, and lower incidence of side effects relative to tricyclic antidepressants medications. However, side effects remain problematic, and include nausea, diarrhea, and tremor. Up to 15% of patients develop sexual side effects, including diminished libido, impotence, or both. SSRIs should not be discontinued abruptly, because withdrawal symptoms may develop.

Serotonin–Norepinephrine Reuptake Inhibitors (SNRIs)

Serotonin–norepinephrine reuptake inhibitors (SNRIs) medications are similar to SSRIs, but they also increase the availability of norepinephrine. The advantages are that they influence both serotonin and norepinephrine, but do not have all the negative side effects of the tricyclic antidepressant medications. However, side effects are sometimes problematic and include nausea, nervousness, diminished appetite, dizziness, and a dry mouth. Although these medications are marketed as causing a lower rate of sexual side effects relative to SSRIs, diminished libido and impotence may be problematic.

Other Antidepressants

The side effects of other antidepressants depend on their mechanism of action. Bupropion, which influences both norepinephrine and dopamine, has been reported to cause seizures in high doses. Other side effects include nervousness, irritability, and insomnia. Mirtazapine, which influences serotonin, norepinephrine, and other brain mechanisms, is much more sedating than are traditional SSRIs and SNRIs. In rare cases, this medication can diminish the body's platelets, white blood cells, and red blood cells. Other side effects include weight gain and diminished libido. Trazodone is an older antidepressant medication that is highly sedating. Because of its sedating effects, trazodone is more often used as a treatment for insomnia. Other side effects include dizziness, dry mouth, and constipation.

Indications in Pain Management

The decision to use an antidepressant medication should be guided by the nature of the patient's pain and any accompanying depression and anxiety. It also is possible to take advantage of some of the side effects with some of these medications. For example, patients who have severe pain and insomnia may benefit from antidepressant medications that cause sedation. Patients with urinary frequency may benefit from antidepressants that cause urinary retention.

In addition to understanding the side-effect profile of these medications, and possibly taking advantage of side effects, antidepressants may be an important medication simply as a treatment for pain. For example, patients with chronic, neuropathic pain may improve functionally following the introduction of an antidepressant medication. Indeed, virtually every antidepressant medication has demonstrated efficacy in treating chronic pain. Only duloxetine (Cymbalta) has received FDA approval for treatment of pain disorders, and this FDA indication is limited to postherpetic neuralgia and diabetic nerve pain. However, it is extremely common for physicians to utilize antidepressant medications in an off-label manner for the treatment of chronic, neuropathic pain.

In addition to the effect of these medications on pain, antidepressant medications are often utilized in treating patients with chronic pain because these patients usually suffer with depression and anxiety. The newer SSRIs and SNRIs are extremely effective in treating both depression and anxiety and, for this reason, they may be an important adjunct in the patient's overall medical treatment. Effective treatment of depression and anxiety is a cornerstone to improving patient function.

COMMONLY PRESCRIBED ANTIDEPRESSANTS: TRICYCLIC ANTIDEPRESSANTS

Table 5.3 lists the tricyclic antidepressants commonly prescribed in the treatment of chronic pain.

Table 5.3
Commonly Prescribed Tricyclic Antidepressants for Chronic Pain

Generic Name	Brand Name	Starting Dose	Maintenance Dose
Amitriptyline	Elavil	10mg at night	10-100mg at night
Desipramine	Norpramin	10mg at night	10-100mg at night
Imipramine	Tofranil	10mg at night	10-100mg at night
Nortriptyline	Pamelor	10mg at night	10-100mg at night

Amitriptyline (Elavil)

Amitriptyline is the best studied of all tricyclic antidepressants in the treatment of pain. Amitriptyline may produce beneficial effects in any type of chronic pain condition. Because amitriptyline is quite sedating, it also effectively treats insomnia. The usual starting dose is 10 mg at night, and this dosage is then increased slowly in 10-mg increments every few weeks, as tolerated and needed. Amitriptyline has more side effects than do most other antidepressant medications, including sedation, weight gain, dizziness, dry mouth, and urinary retention.

Desipramine (Norpramin)

Desipramine has fewer side effects than does amitriptyline, and it may be more beneficial in alleviating underlying anxiety. The usual starting dose is 10 mg at night, and this dose is then increased in 10-mg increments every few weeks, as tolerated and needed.

Imipramine (Tofranil)

Like amitriptyline, imipramine is very effective in helping to alleviate pain. It has similar side effects, including sedation, weight gain, dizziness, dry mouth, and urinary retention. The usual starting dose is 10 mg at night, and this dose is increased in 10-mg increments every few weeks, as tolerated and needed.

Nortriptyline (Pamelor)

Nortriptyline has fewer side effects than does amitriptyline and, for this reason, may be preferable for patients who cannot tolerate amitriptyline.

The usual starting dose is 10 mg at night, and this dose can be increased in 10-mg increments every few weeks, as tolerated and needed.

SELECTIVE SEROTONIN REUPTAKE INHIBITORS

Table 5.4 lists the SSRIs commonly prescribed in the treatment of chronic pain.

TABLE 5.4
Commonly Prescribed Selective Serotonin Reuptake Inhibitors for Chronic Pain

GENERIC NAME	BRAND NAME	STARTING DOSE	MAINTENANCE DOSE
Citalopram	Celexa	20mg daily	20-60mg daily
Fluoxetine	Prozac	20mg daily	20-80mg daily
Paroxetine	Paxil, Paxil CR	10-20mg daily	10-60mg daily
Sertraline	Zoloft	25mg daily	25-200mg daily

Citalopram (Celexa)

Citalopram is indicated for the treatment of depression but may be used off-label to treat anxiety and pain. Side effects are similar to those of all other SSRIs. The usual starting dose is 20 mg daily, and this dose is then increased in 20-mg increments every 1 to 2 weeks, as tolerated and needed. The maximum dose is 60 mg per day.

Fluoxetine (Prozac)

Fluoxetine was introduced in 1987, and it revolutionized the treatment of depression. It is indicated for the treatment of depression, manic depressive disorder, obsessive-compulsive disorder, and bulimia. Its side effects are similar to those of other SSRIs. The recommended starting dose is 20 mg daily, and this dose may be increased in 10-mg to 20-mg increments every 1 to few weeks, as tolerated and needed. The maximum dose is 80 mg per day.

Paroxetine (Paxil, Paxil CR)

Paroxetine is indicated for the treatment of depression and obsessive-compulsive disorder, and it is also utilized off-label to treat anxiety and chronic pain. Its side effects are similar to those of other SSRIs. The usual starting dose is 10 mg to 20 mg per day, and this dose may be increased in 10-mg to 20-mg increments every 1 to few weeks, as tolerated and needed. The maximum dose is 60 mg per day.

Sertraline (Zoloft)

Sertraline is indicated for treatment of depression and obsessive com-pulsive disorder. It is used off-label to treat anxiety and chronic pain. Its side effects are similar to those of other SSRIs. The usual starting dose is 25 mg daily, and this dose is increased in 25-mg increments every 1 to few weeks, as tolerated and needed. The maximum dose is 200 mg per day.

SEROTONIN-NOREPINEPHRINE REUPTAKE INHIBITORS

Table 5.5 lists the SNRIs commonly prescribed in the treatment of chron-ic pain.

TABLE 5.5
Commonly Prescribed Serotonin-Norepinephrine Reuptake Inhibitors for Chronic Pain

GENERIC NAME	BRAND NAME	STARTING DOSE	MAINTENANCE DOSE
Duloxetine	Cymbalta	20-40mg daily	60-120mg, in 2 divided doses
Venlafaxine	Effexor, Effexor XR	37.5mg daily	75-300mg daily

Duloxetine (Cymbalta)

Duloxetine is unique in that it is not only indicated for the treatment of depression, but also in the treatment of diabetic nerve pain and postherpet-ic neuralgia. It is also commonly utilized to treat other chronic pain condi-tions. Side effects are similar to those of the SNRIs as discussed above. The usual starting dose is 20 mg to 40 mg per day. This dosage is then increased in 20-mg to 40-mg increments, as tolerated and needed, to a maximum dose of 60 mg twice daily.

Venlafaxine (Effexor, Effexor XR)

Venlafaxine is indicated in the treatment of depression and anxiety, and is commonly used off-label to treat chronic pain. Its side effects are similar to those of other SNRIs. The usual starting dose is 37.5 mg in an extended-release form once daily, and this dosage is then increased in 37.5-mg weekly increments, as tolerated and needed, to a maximum dose of 300 mg per day.

OTHER ANTIDEPRESSANTS

Table 5.6 lists other antidepressants commonly prescribed in the treatment of chronic pain.

TABLE 5.6
Other Commonly Prescribed Antidepressants for Chronic Pain

GENERIC NAME	BRAND NAME	STARTING DOSE	MAINTENANCE DOSE
Bupropion	Wellbutrin SR/XL, Zyban	150mg daily	300-600mg daily, in 2 doses for SR, 1 dose for XL
Mirtazapine	Remeron	15mg at night	15-60mg at night
Trazodone	Desyrel	50mg at night	50-600 mg at night

Bupropion (Wellbutrin SR/XL, Zyban)

Bupropion influences both norepinephrine and dopamine availability. Because the dopamine brain pathways are frequently involved in our craving behavior, bupropion is used not only for depression, but also for nicotine addiction. It also is used as an adjunct when treating patients with chronic pain. Restlessness is a more common side effect of bupropion. The normal starting dose is 150 mg per day, and this dosage may be increased in 75-mg to 150-mg increments every 1 to few weeks, as tolerated and needed, to a maximum dose of 600 mg per day.

Mirtazapine (Remeron)

Mirtazapine influences both serotonin and norepinephrine pathways, and it has powerful sedating side effects. It is indicated in the treatment of depression and anxiety, and it is also used as an adjunct in treating chronic pain. Typically, mirtazapine only is utilized at night. It is begun at 15 mg, and increased in 15-mg increments every 1 to few weeks, as tolerated and needed, to a maximum dose of 60 mg per day.

Trazodone (Desyrel)

Trazodone is an older antidepressant medication that is now more commonly used to treat insomnia. In treating chronic pain, its effects on insomnia are very important, and it also may have some independent pain-relieving qualities. The usual starting dose is 50 mg at night, and this dosage is increased in 50-mg to 150-mg increments every 1 to few weeks, as tolerated and needed, to a maximum dose of 600 mg per day.

ANTICONVULSANTS

How They Work

Anticonvulsant medications are used to treat epilepsy and other seizure disorders. From a simplistic point of view, anticonvulsants work by preventing nerve cell hyperexcitability. Seizures are a result of a localized or generalized process within the brain, in which groups of cells suddenly begin to fire in an uncontrolled manner. This leads to any combination of shaking of the limbs, changes in speech, changes in level of consciousness, and in severe cases, prolonged shaking with loss of consciousness.

Within the cells of the brain, various channels allow various substances such as sodium, potassium, or calcium to enter into or to leave the cell. When these elements come into or out of the cell, the excitability of the cell can change. Many of the anticonvulsants work by blocking sodium or calcium channels. Others influence the availability of GABA, which is a neurochemical that influences not only brain excitability, but also muscle spasticity.

Years ago, it was discovered that some anticonvulsants are extremely effective in treating a specific pain disorder called *trigeminal neuralgia*. This is a neuropathic pain condition in which extreme, electric shock–like pain is experienced within the face. Once it was discovered that anticonvulsants were effective in treating trigeminal neuralgia, it became common to utilize these medications in treating other pain conditions, including diabetic nerve pain, postherpetic neuralgia, and other chronic neuropathic pain conditions. Although only gabapentin and pregabalin have received formal FDA approval for treating certain pain conditions, it is common to utilize a wide variety of anticonvulsant medications to treat chronic, neuropathic pain.

Side Effects

The side effects of anticonvulsants depend on the particular drug utilized. In general, most of these medications can cause some sedation and dizziness. Because side effects can vary widely depending on the type of anticonvulsant utilized, more specific side effects are described in each of the sections following.

Indications in Pain Management

Anticonvulsants have revolutionized the pharmacology of pain management. It is extremely common for patients with chronic, neuropathic pain to be treated with an anticonvulsant. Even though most of these medications are used off-label, their clinical efficacy is quite well established in the medical literature. Chronic neuropathic pain can be considered a hyperexcitable state both within the brain and the spinal cord. Because anticonvulsants stabilize cell hyperexcitability, they can stabilize the pain pathways. They are used in a wide variety of pain disorders, ranging from peripheral nerve pain to chronic low back pain to chronic headache.

Patients may respond quite differently to the various anticonvulsants. Therefore, if a patient suffers with chronic pain and does not respond to one anticonvulsant, another may be tried. Anticonvulsants are not a stand-alone treatment, but should be part of multidisciplinary treatment, including the use of other medications, behavioral strategies, group therapy, physical therapy, and psychological therapy.

COMMONLY PRESCRIBED ANTICONVULSANTS

Table 5.7 lists the anticonvulsants commonly prescribed in the treatment of chronic pain.

TABLE 5.7
Commonly Prescribed Anticonvulsants for Chronic Pain

GENERIC NAME	BRAND NAME	STARTING DOSE	MAINTENANCE DOSE
Carbamazepine	Carbatrol, Tegretol, Tegretol XL	100mg 1-2 times daily	400-1600mg daily, in 2-4 divided doses
Gabapentin	Neurontin	100mg 1-3 times daily	600-4000mg daily, in 3-4 divided doses
Lamotrigine	Lamictal	25mg 1-2 times daily	100-200mg twice daily
Oxcarbazepine	Trileptal	75-150mg 1-2 times daily	600-2400mg daily, in 2 divided doses
Pregabalin	Lyrica	25-50mg 2-3 times daily	150mg twice daily
Topiramate	Topamax	25-50mg at night	100-400mg daily, in 1-2 doses
Valproic Acid	Depakene, Depakote SR/ER	250mg once daily	500-2000mg daily, in 1-2 divided doses
Zonisamide	Zonegran	25-100mg at night	100-600mg at night

Carbamazepine (Carbatrol, Tegretol, Tegretol XL)

Carbamazepine is an older anticonvulsant that has been demonstrated in many studies to be a highly effective treatment for trigeminal neuralgia and diabetic nerve pain. In general, patients with electric shock–like pain, burning pain, or lancinating pain may benefit from treatment with carbamazepine. Side effects include sedation, dizziness, and disequilibrium. Patients must undergo monitoring of their blood count, because carbamazepine can lower the white blood cell count. Some patients develop a lowering of their blood sodium level, and this must be monitored as well. The usual starting dose is 100 mg one to two times daily, and this dosage is increased in 100-mg to 200-mg weekly increments, as tolerated and needed, to a maximum dose of 1,600 mg per day.

Gabapentin (Neurontin)

Just as carbamazepine helped to revolutionize pain management for pain conditions such as trigeminal neuralgia and diabetic nerve pain, gabapentin has expanded this revolution into a wide variety of chronic pain disorders.

Indeed, it is the combination of gabapentin's efficacy and low side effect profile that has paved the way for physicians to become comfortable in using anticonvulsants when treating patients with chronic pain. Gabapentin increases the availability of the brain chemical GABA, and it also influences the manner in which calcium enters into a cell.

Its side effects include dizziness, sedation, and weight gain, but patients often develop tolerance to these side effects. The normal starting dose is 100 mg to 300 mg per day, and the dosage is increased in 100-mg to 300-mg weekly increments, as tolerated and needed. Generally speaking, gabapentin must be taken three to four times daily. In patients with severe, chronic neuropathic pain, the dosage may be increased to 4,000 mg per day.

Lamotrigine (Lamictal)

Lamotrigine works by influencing the manner in which sodium enters the cell, and it also suppresses a highly excitable brain chemical called *glutamate*. Lamotrigine must be started very slowly, because a high incidence of rash occurs within the first several weeks of use. This rash can become quite serious and may even require hospitalization. Side effects otherwise include dizziness and somnolence, but over the long term, lamotrigine is a very well-tolerated anticonvulsant. It often is used for patients who complain of burning, lancinating, or electric shock–like pain. The initial starting dose is 25 mg one to two times daily. This dosage is increased very slowly over the first 5 weeks to a target dose of 100 mg twice daily. If patients have not developed a skin rash, the dosage can then be increased further to a maximum of 200 mg twice daily.

Oxcarbazepine (Trileptal)

Oxcarbazepine is somewhat similar to carbamazepine, in that it also influences the sodium availability within a cell. Its side effects include somnolence, dizziness, and lowering of the blood sodium level. Thus, blood tests must be obtained to monitor the blood sodium. Oxcarbazepine is used more commonly in patients who complain of burning, electric shock–like, or lancinating pain. The normal starting dose is 150 mg per day, and this dosage is increased in 150-mg to 300-mg weekly increments, as tolerated and needed, to a maximum dose of 2,400 mg per day.

Pregabalin (Lyrica)

Pregabalin is a newer anticonvulsant that influences GABA and calcium entry within a cell. Pregabalin has FDA approval for the treatment of diabetic nerve pain and postherpetic neuralgia, but it is also used off-label for other chronic pain conditions. Side effects include dizziness, sedation, dry mouth, and weight gain. The usual starting dose is 25 mg to 50 mg two to three times daily, and this dosage is increased in 50-mg weekly increments, as tolerated and needed, to a maximum dose of 300 mg per day.

Topiramate (Topamax)

Topiramate influences the availability of both sodium and GABA entry into a cell. Topiramate has FDA approval for the treatment of migraine, and it is commonly used off-label to treat other chronic neuropathic pain conditions. Its side effects include sedation and dizziness. A higher incident of kidney stones occurs in patients who use topiramate. Many patients complain of an uncomfortable tingling sensation in their hands and feet, and this tingling sensation is often relieved by the ingestion of vitamin C 500 mg daily and one banana daily. Anorexia and weight loss are common with topiramate. The usual starting dose is 25 mg to 50 mg at night; this dosage is then increased in 25-mg to 50-mg weekly increments, as tolerated and needed, to a maximum dosage of 400 mg per day.

Valproic Acid (Depakene, Depakote SR/ER)

Valproic acid influences the availability of both sodium and GABA entry into a cell. Valproic acid is used more commonly in the treatment of chronic migraine and other headache conditions, although it has been used in some neuropathic pain conditions as well. Common side effects include dizziness, somnolence, and gastrointestinal upset. The blood and platelet count must be monitored with valproic acid use because some patients develop a reduction in their platelet count. Liver enzymes also must be monitored in patients who take this medication. Women of menstrual age may develop ovarian and kidney cysts. The normal starting dose is 250 mg daily, and this dose can be increased in 250-mg weekly increments, as tolerated and needed, to a maximum dose of 2,000 mg per day.

Zonisamide (Zonegran)

Zonisamide influences both sodium and calcium entry into the cell, as well as the availability of GABA. Side effects include dizziness, gait imbalance, and diminished appetite. Kidney stones are more common in patients who utilize zonisamide. The initial starting dose is 100 mg at night, and this dosage can be increased in 100-mg weekly increments, as tolerated and needed, to a maximum dose of 600 mg per day.

TOPICAL ANALGESICS

Topical analgesics generally are packaged as a cream or as a self-adhesive patch. The most well-studied topical analgesic is a 5% lidocaine patch (Lidoderm). Topical analgesics allow a well-defined, painful area to be treated by becoming anesthetized. Topical analgesics are useful for localized muscle spasm or pain, but generally are ineffective for low back pain caused by a herniated disc or one of the deep muscles of the spine. Side effects are few and generally include a localized rash. Capsaicin, which is more often used for chronic nerve pain, has little role in the treatment of other low back conditions.

CORTICOSTEROIDS

Corticosteroids (glucocorticosteroids) can be very effective for the acute management of severe low back pain or sciatica, especially from a herniated lumbar disc. Corticosteroids are not *anabolic steroids*. Anabolic steroids most often are used illegally by athletes to enhance muscle strength and endurance. Corticosteroids are very potent anti-inflammatory medications and, in situations such as an acute lumbar disc herniation, can lead to very effective reduction in associated nerve root and regional swelling. Corticosteroids most often are prescribed as a pulse therapy, generally over a period of 5 to 10 days. In *pulse therapy*, the treatment begins with a moderate to high dose of corticosteroid medication, and the dose is then decreased daily. Corticosteroids often can be given by way of injection, which is discussed in Chapter 6.

The long-term use of corticosteroids is reserved for rheumatologic conditions such as rheumatoid arthritis. Several serious side effects are associated with the long-term use of corticosteroids, including immune dysfunction, weakening of the bones, and muscle atrophy.

SUMMARY POINTS

- The FDA approves the marketing of medications for specific indications. However, it is commonplace for physicians to prescribe a medication "off-label," which means for conditions that have not been approved by the FDA.
- Nonsteroidal anti-inflammatory drugs are divided into COX-1 and COX-2 inhibitors. They are useful in treating acute pain.
- Muscle relaxants reduce the painful muscle spasm that often accompanies acute pain.
- Narcotic analgesics are the most potent analgesic prescription medication. They are utilized in the treatment of moderate to severe pain.
- Antidepressant medications benefit patients with chronic pain both by treating the underlying depression and anxiety of chronic pain, and by modifying the pain pathways.
- Anticonvulsant medications benefit patients with chronic pain by modifying the pain pathways.

CHAPTER 6

Nonsurgical Treatments

HANDS-ON TREATMENT AND EXERCISE

Physical Therapy

Physical therapy is often the first line of treatment for patients who suffer with low back pain, especially if their first contact has been with an internist, primary care physician, or orthopedic surgeon. Physical therapy treatment can include modalities, hands-on massage and manipulation, and therapeutic exercises.

Physical therapy modalites include, but are not limited to, the application of ice, ultrasound (Figure 6.1), electrical stimulation (Figure 6.2), heat, and topical creams. Some physical therapists are specialized in spinal manipulation, and others specialize in more intuitive techniques such as craniosacral technique and myofascial release, which are described below. These latter two techniques require extensive one-on-one time, at least 30 to 60 minutes, and the therapist is constantly monitoring the patient's physical and emotional response to the treatment.

Therapeutic exercises range from the most simplistic of low back exercises to progressive spinal stabilization techniques and the use of specialized weight machines. Too often, patients enter a physical therapy facility, receive a cursory treatment with one modality or another, undergo simple stretching and strengthening exercises, and are then provided cookbook exercises to perform. Although this may work for uncomplicated low back pain, it is generally ineffective for more complicated or chronic low back conditions.

For more complicated or chronic cases, specialized care is required. This specialized care includes more extensive one-on-one manual work, by way of either manipulation, myofascial release, craniosacral technique,

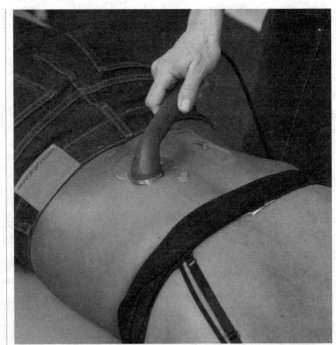

Figure 6.1
Ultrasound treatment.

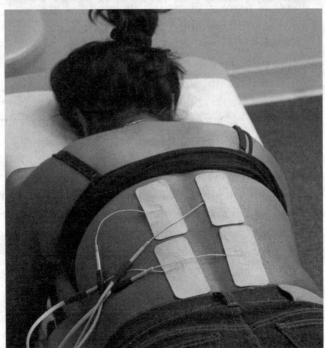

Figure 6.2
Treatment with electrical stimulation.

Feldenkrais method, or Alexander technique, coupled with a much more specialized progressive exercise and spine stabilization protocol. When a physical therapy facility depends on reimbursement based on the number of patients treated per hour, the facility may not provide specialized one-on-one care.

Lumbar stabilization is an exercise program designed to strengthen spinal support muscles while achieving a "neutral spine" position. The patient learns to rely on the body's proprioception or feedback system to increase awareness of spine and other joint position (Figure 6.3). Often, exercises include the use of a large air-filled ball, and the ongoing focus is balance and strength. Lumbar stabilization exercises cannot simply be learned from a book; the therapist must constantly ensure proper posture, position, and patient readiness for progression in such exercises (Figure 6.4).

Craniosacral therapy is an intuitive, hands-on technique practiced by specialized physical therapists, massage therapists, and chiropractors. Craniosacral therapists gently manipulate the soft tissue and bones of the head, down the spine, and into the sacral and pelvic region. The treatment is quite relaxing, and the therapist's work theoretically helps to ensure proper spinal fluid flow. Intuition in this case means that the therapist is not simply following a set pattern, but is monitoring the patient's physical and emotional responses to each phase of treatment (Figure 6.5).

Myofascial release is a technique that eases pressure in the fibrous bands of connective tissue that encase muscles and organs throughout the body. The theory of myofascial release is that injury or illness leads to scarring or impediment of movement in the connective tissue network, thereby causing dysfunction and pain. Restoration of movement is obtained through the therapist's gentle and intuitive myofascial release techniques (Figure 6.6).

The *Alexander technique* is a method whose aim is to change movement habits that are associated with neuromuscular dysfunction. The Alexander technique is not a series of exercises, but rather a focus of mind and body re-education. Stress reduction and freedom of movement are the cornerstones of this technique.

The *Feldenkrais method* is a physical therapy technique whose goal is to improve posture, coordination, and flexibility. Through a series of postures, patterns of inefficiency can be improved, while repressed feelings can be rediscovered.

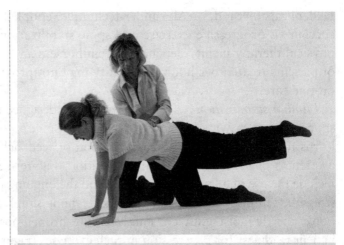

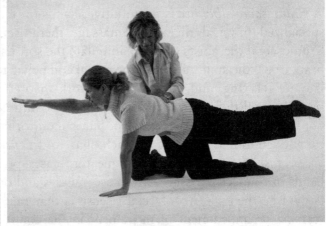

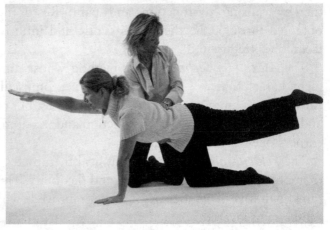

FIGURE 6.3
Sequential photographs demonstrating lumbar stabilization exercises, with the therapist guiding the patient in body position and awareness.

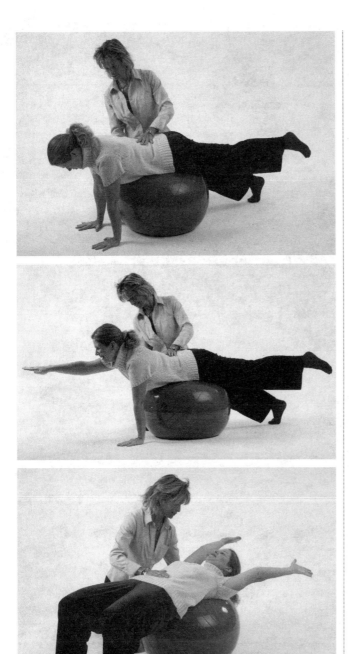

FIGURE 6.4
*Sequential
photographs
demonstrating the
interplay between
physical therapist and
patient utilizing an air-
filled ball for lumbar
stabilization exercises.*

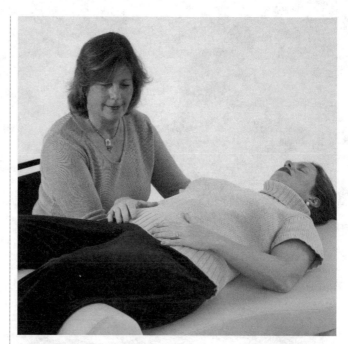

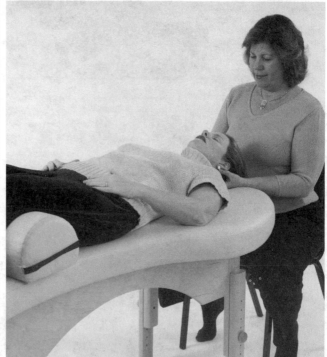

FIGURE 6.5
*Craniosacral
technique.*

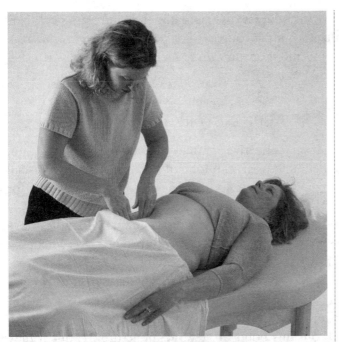

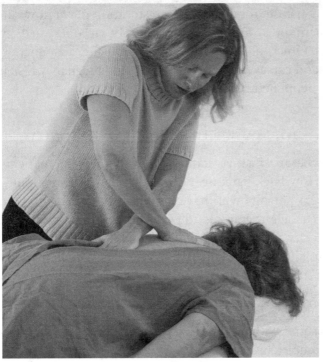

FIGURE 6.6
*Different myofascial
release techniques.*

The physical therapy techniques discussed above require physical therapists to take specialized training courses. For patients with chronic back pain, it is worth the time and monetary investment to work with such specialized therapists.

ACUPUNCTURE

Acupuncture can be a very effective strategy for acute low back pain, because the skilled acupuncturist can obtain an excellent myofascial release in an area of regional muscle spasm. The effect of acupuncture for more chronic low back conditions is less apparent. Acupuncture is only somewhat effective for chronic pain; although a number of studies have demonstrated some efficacy, the evidence does not provide overwhelming support for acupuncture as a stand-alone treatment.

The Chinese developed a system of meridian points, which in essence define areas of energy flow (*chi*). A skilled acupuncturist treats a patient based on his perception of *chi* flow, and uses the acupuncture needle to restore *chi* balance. From this point of view, acupuncture treatment may be required over a long period of time, because restoration of *chi* flow can take weeks and even months, and generally must be accompanied by other lifestyle changes. Other than localized pain or bruising, acupuncture is very well tolerated and can even be used safely during pregnancy, when practiced by a skilled acupuncturist (Figure 6.7).

MASSAGE THERAPY

Massage therapy can be an effective stand-alone treatment for patients who suffer with acute low back pain, or it can be used as part of a multidisciplinary approach in patients who have chronic low back pain. One important aspect of massage therapy is touch. Massage therapists learn specialized techniques that require utilizing their hands in a skilled and professional manner to allow the body to relax. Sometimes touch involves a kneading technique that helps to release muscle spasm (Figure 6.8). Other times, touch may be barely perceptible, with the purpose of guiding the patient to release or relax a certain area of the body.

Some patients who suffer with chronic low back pain have limited experience of being in a completely relaxed state while being touched. This is

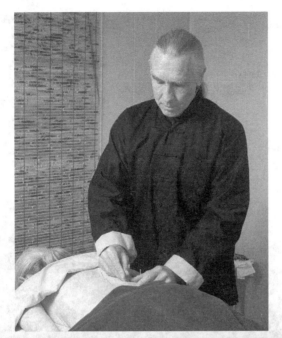

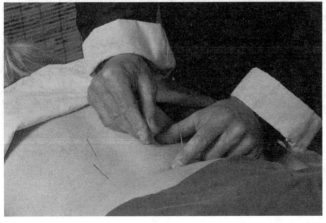

FIGURE 6.7
*Acupuncture
treatment.*

because they have developed several maladaptive strategies over time and may be fearful of being touched while lying in a completely relaxed and vulnerable position. Indeed, it is not uncommon for patients with chronic neuropathic pain to develop a cathartic, emotional response while undergoing massage therapy. This sudden emotional release likely

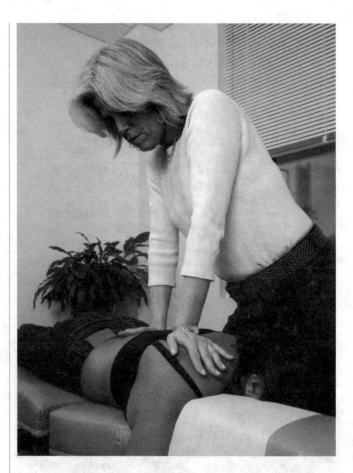

FIGURE 6.8
Kneading technique in massage therapy.

occurs because the patient is no longer in a guarded position, and he may then develop a sudden insight into certain emotions that are intertwined with chronic pain.

SPINAL MANIPULATION

Spinal manipulation is a technique that can be performed by physical therapists, chiropractors, osteopathic physicians, or others who have received specialty training. Although some chiropractors claim that they are the only clinicians who have specialty training in spinal manipulation, this simply is not the case. However, it should be noted that chiropractors rely more on spinal manipulation as a means of treatment, relative to physical therapists and osteopathic physicians. In spinal manipulation, the practitioner places the patient in a certain position, then through either prolonged pressure or a sudden thrust movement, the patient's spinal alignment is adjusted (Figure 6.9).

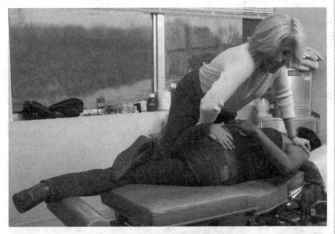

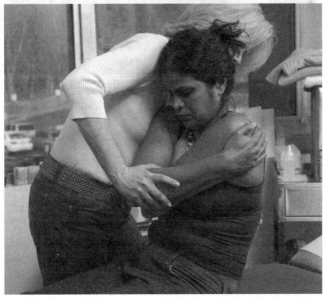

FIGURE 6.9
Spinal manipulation utilizing a sudden thrust movement (above) and prolonged pressure (below).

Spinal manipulation is a very effective treatment for the management of acute back pain, and sometimes it may be effective in patients with more chronic pain. The difficulty with spinal manipulation in chronic pain patients is that such patients have often developed several maladaptive strategies that will simply not respond to acute manipulation. Although acute manipulation may be immediately helpful, the maladaptive physiologic or musculoskeletal response often recurs after treatment is completed. Some specialists in spinal manipulation argue that treatment is required for a prolonged period of time, but it is more reasonable to say that if a spinal manipulation is ineffective within a few weeks, another treatment strategy should be sought.

For uncomplicated low back pain, patients generally prefer spinal manipulation to other treatment strategies. This is likely because of its effectiveness and direct, hands-on approach. Spinal manipulation techniques do not restore a disc into its normal place. Rather, spinal manipulation helps to restore balance in the spine and, when such a balance is achieved, the body's innate healing response may occur more readily.

BIOFEEDBACK

Biofeedback is an effective treatment for patients who have a propensity to muscle spasm, or for patients who have anxiety associated with chronic pain. Biofeedback is not a first-line treatment for acute low back pain.

Biofeedback is performed by attaching the patient to specialized sensors that relay signals to a computerized machine. The sensors may detect muscle spasm or temperature and, through constant feedback signals from the computerized machine, the patient learns to change the signals. A practitioner guides the patient throughout this process.

In some patients, specific environmental or emotional triggers lead to an augmentation of their pain response. If the patient can learn to recognize such triggers and prevent the body's reflex response to such triggers, then biofeedback becomes especially useful as an adjunct in chronic pain management. Once patients learn biofeedback with a trained specialist, they can practice these techniques at home, thereby perfecting the ability to diminish anxiety-driven pain responses (Figure 6.10).

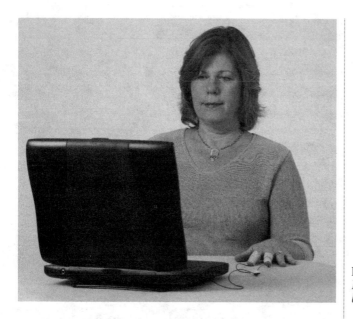

FIGURE 6.10
*Patient practicing
biofeedback.*

RELAXATION AND MEDITATION

Relaxation and meditation techniques are vastly underutilized in the treatment of both acute and chronic low back pain. Several studies have demonstrated the effectiveness of meditative techniques in altering the body's physiologic response, especially with regard to chronic pain.

A simple form of meditation can be performed when the patient is either sitting in a firm, comfortable chair, or sitting or reclining on the floor. The patient breathes comfortably and slowly through the nose, trying to breathe deeply into the umbilicus region, and not shallowly into the chest (Figure 6.11). He then tries to focus more and more on breathing alone, gently letting go of other thoughts and distractions. This is often quite difficult initially, and some people prefer to focus on a relaxing thought or image.

In addition to diminishing the amplitude of a heightened physiologic response, meditation may

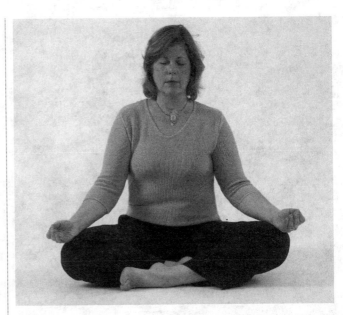

FIGURE 6.11
A meditation pose.

also help a patient to develop insight into his condition. Even at a simplistic level, a patient who has developed low back pain may have done so in the setting of considerable stress. However, the patient may not have an appreciation of the relationship between stress and the low back pain incident. During meditation, the individual transcends the normal workaday world and becomes more focused on simple breathing and being. If this state of mind is achieved, then the patient may begin to appreciate how stress and its associated physiologic response can negatively impact the body.

EXERCISES

Many exercises have a therapeutic role in the treatment of both acute and chronic low back pain. Patients with both acute and chronic low back pain require exercise, although generally speaking, this should be done under the guidance of the treating clinician.

Numerous exercises and breathing techniques may benefit patients with low back pain. Only a few are described below but, in general, exercises that require attention to breathing and balance often benefit the low back.

Walking is an often-overlooked therapeutic exercise. Walking develops the paraspinal, gluteal, and leg muscles, all of which are important in helping to stabilize the spine. Walking also can have a therapeutic benefit from a cardiovascular and aerobic point of view.

Yoga is an ancient exercise that employs breathing techniques and postures, generally from a reclining or seated position. In essence, using yoga, patients learn to work with their breath and to understand movement while breathing. Too often, exercise is performed in such a manner that the body is stressed without any feedback or awareness on the part of the person exercising. Even with yoga, some patients try to achieve postures while forgetting to work within the limits of their breathing, and this can lead to injury as well. For patients with low back problems, yoga should be started once they have received clearance from their treating clinician. Yoga can be physically demanding; long term, it is an extraordinarily effective exercise for spine stabilization (Figure 6.12).

T'ai chi is an ancient exercise that is generally performed from a standing position. T'ai chi requires an extraordinary sense of balance and centering, and it also utilizes meditative breathing. Initially, t'ai chi may seem complicated because many different dance-like movements must be memorized. Over the long term, however, the practitioner of t'ai chi becomes more intuitively aware of his body, and this is extremely important for patients who have developed chronic musculoskeletal maladaptation (Figure 6.13).

Chi gong is a type of meditative breathing in which the entire body is used to obtain deep, slow breaths. Chi gong can be performed from a standing or sitting position, and it requires less movement than does t'ai chi (Figure 6.14).

Pilates has become a relatively recent popular form of exercise. Pilates generally is performed from a reclining position. Under proper supervision, Pilates ultimately strengthens the core musculature that is so important in spine stabilization. Like yoga, patients who suffer from a low back condition should begin Pilates after they have received clearance from their treating clinician (Figure 6.15).

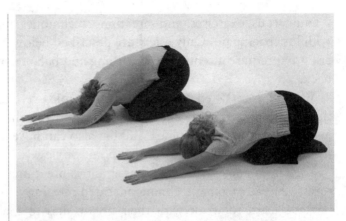

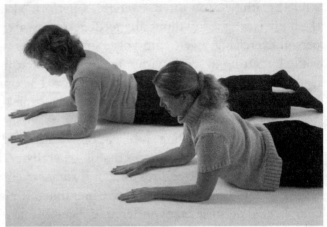

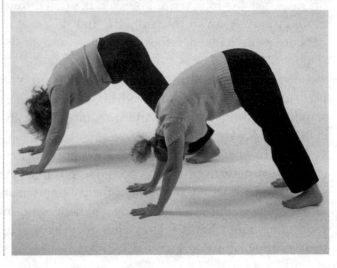

FIGURE 6.12
Various yoga postures.

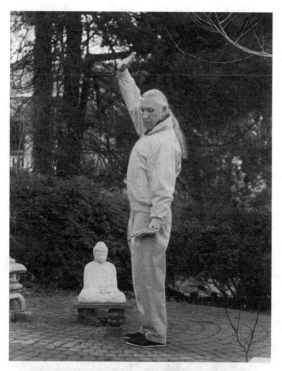

FIGURE 6.13
The meditative balance of t'ai chi.

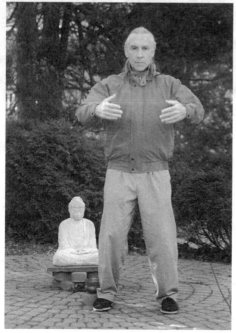

FIGURE 6.14
Chi gong breathing.

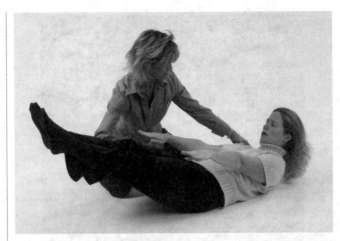

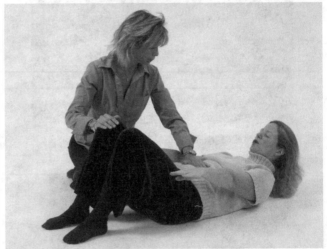

FIGURE 6.15
Interplay between instructor and client with Pilates exercises.

Exercise can be extremely effective in promoting the health of the body in general and the low back in particular. All exercise requires careful attention to the body's mechanics and to the mind–body continuum. Exercise is also an extremely effective form of stress release; this in and of itself may be one of its most salient features. As with the more specific exercises described in the preceding sections, a general exercise program should be started following clearance from the patient's clinician.

THERAPEUTIC INJECTIONS

Trigger-Point Injections

Trigger-point injections are relatively superficial injections of a medication such as lidocaine or corticosteroid, or with a glucose solution (Figure 6.16). Pain anesthesiologists, physiatrists, orthope-

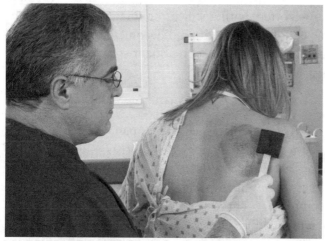

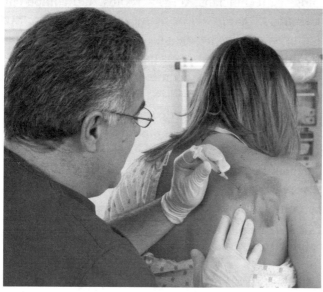

FIGURE 6.16
A patient undergoing trigger-point injections.

dic surgeons, rheumatologists, and neurologists most commonly treat with trigger-point injections. The purpose of these injections is to obtain a regional area of relative anesthesia in general, and to reduce muscle spasm in particular. Some physicians utilize deeper trigger-point injections into the ligament in an attempt to shrink the ligament (*prolotherapy*). The effectiveness of this latter technique is questionable.

Trigger-point injections generally are not used as a stand-alone treatment. They can be a very effective strategy in helping to break a cycle of muscle spasm or regional pain, but such treatment should be accompanied by manual therapy, often with medication management as well. Often, breaking one aspect of the cycle of pain becomes an effective strategy, especially when combined with other treatment strategies.

Epidural Injections

Epidural injections usually are performed by a pain anesthesiologist, although orthopedics surgeons, neurologists, physiatrists and radiologists also may receive training in this procedure. Epidural injections should be performed in an ambulatory surgical or similar setting, with x-ray fluoroscopy guidance. Ambulatory surgery centers are designed so that patients can undergo a procedure or surgery and return home the same day. Nurses, anesthesiologists, technicians, surgery rooms, and equipment are the norm in such centers. *X-ray fluoroscopy* is a movable x-ray machine that a physician uses to guide needle placement.

To receive an epidural injection, the patient is generally in a prone position (Figure 6.17). If this position is too uncomfortable, the patient may be seated. The area of the spine to be injected is washed and draped in a sterile manner, and a local anesthetic is provided in the area to be injected. In addition, some patients receive intravenous sedation to minimize any associated anxiety. The physician then uses a spinal needle to enter the epidural space, which is outside of the spinal canal (Figure 6.18). Medication then is delivered by way of a catheter. The most commonly used medications are a combination of an anesthetic such as Marcaine and a corticosteroid such as Depo-Medrol (see Chapter 5). The procedure is usually essentially painless.

Epidural injections are indicated in patients who suffer with lumbar disc herniations or lumbar stenosis; both of these conditions are discussed in

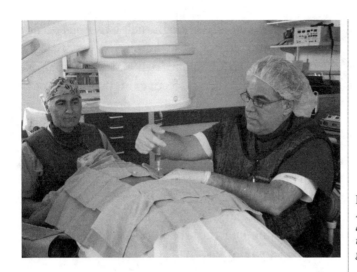

FIGURE 6.17
A patient undergoing an epidural injection with fluoroscopic guidance.

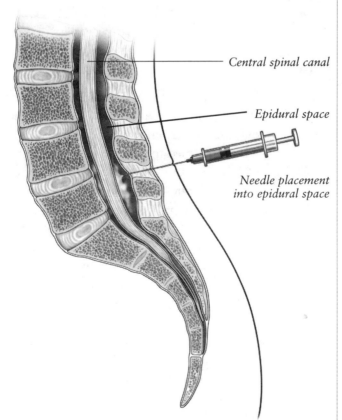

Central spinal canal

Epidural space

Needle placement into epidural space

FIGURE 6.18
The position of the spinal needle during an epidural injection.

subsequent chapters. Although such injections do not correct the underlying disc herniation or stenosis, they lead to a reduction in regional inflammation, and can be extremely effective in providing pain relief. Once pain relief is obtained, a prudent program of rehabilitation should be started. In some patients with chronic low back conditions, epidural corticosteroids can be safely utilized every 4 to 6 months. If such injections are provided more frequently, then the side effects of corticosteroids can develop, which include diminished immune function, bone loss, and muscle atrophy.

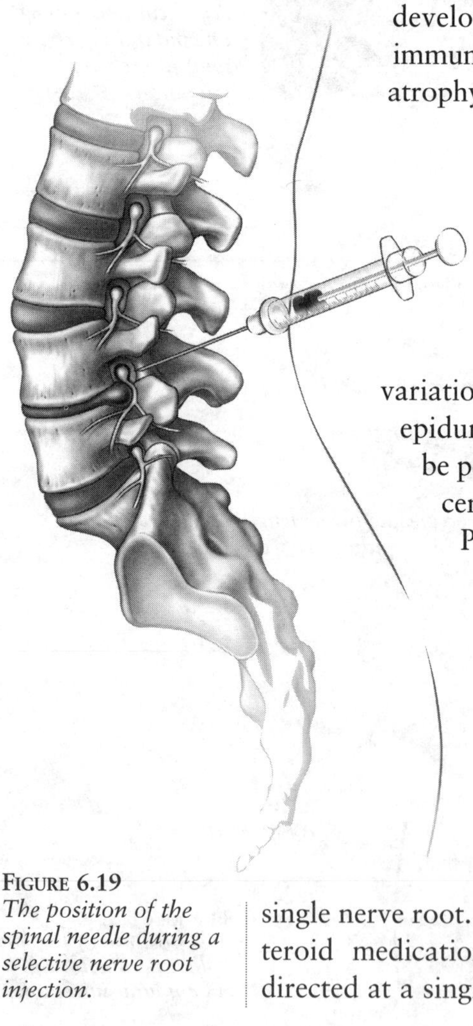

Selective Nerve Root Injection (Trans-Foraminal Injection)

A selective nerve root injection is a variation of the epidural injection. Like an epidural injection, this procedure should be performed in an ambulatory surgery center using fluoroscopic guidance. Pain anesthesiologists most commonly provide selective nerve root injections, but physiatrists, orthopedic surgeons, radiologists, and neurologists may also receive training in this technique. In selective nerve root injections, the foramen (side canal) is selectively entered and medication is delivered along a single nerve root. Using this technique, less corticosteroid medication is utilized, and medication is directed at a single level (Figure 6.19).

FIGURE 6.19
The position of the spinal needle during a selective nerve root injection.

Selective nerve root injections are especially use-ful for patients who have a well-defined nerve root entrapment, either as result of a lumbar disc hernia-tion or as a result of spinal stenosis. Selective nerve root injections are sometimes quite effective in breaking the cycle of radiating leg pain, thereby allowing the opportunity to begin rehabilitation. In some patients, selective nerve root injections, like epidural injections, are given every 4 to 6 months. The procedure should be essentially painless.

Facet Injections

Facet injections are therapeutic injections somewhat similar to epidural injections in that they also are delivered by a pain anesthesi-ologist or another physi-cian who has received specialty training in therapeutic injections. Unlike epidural injec-tions and selective nerve root injections, the patient receives a localized injection of medication into the facet joint (Figure 6.20). Several facet joints can be treated concomi-tantly. Facet pain is explained in detail in Chapter 12.

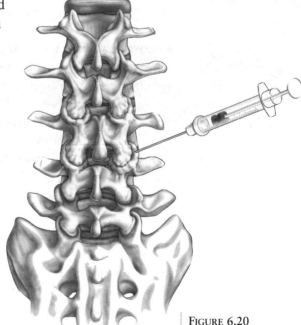

Facet injections should be performed under x-ray fluoroscopic guidance in an ambulato-

FIGURE 6.20
The placement of spinal needle into the facet joint.

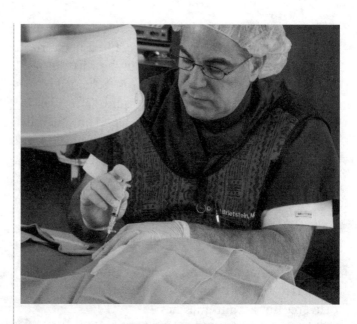

FIGURE 6.21
A patient undergoing a facet injection with fluoroscopic guidance.

ry surgery center (Figure 6.21). These injections are an effective management strategy for patients who have degenerative lumbar spine conditions, lumbar stenosis, or spinal instability. In all these conditions, the facet joint has become transformed into a weight-bearing structure, and becomes chronically inflamed and irritated. Like epidurals, facet injections should be essentially painless. These injections can help break the cycle of pain, thereby allowing the patient to begin a rehabilitation program.

In some patients, facet injections are extremely effective, but the pain recurs weeks to months following the procedure. In such patients, a *rhizotomy* may be considered. Unlike facet injections, a rhizotomy procedure utilizes an electrical or chemical technique to deaden the nerve within the facet joint. This leads to more long-lasting pain relief in appropriate patients. As with facet injections, rhizotomy procedures should be followed by progressive rehabilitation. Facet injections and rhizotomy procedures are essentially painless.

Intradiscal Electrothermal Therapy

Intradiscal electrothermal therapy (IDET) is a relatively new treatment for patients who have low back pain that is secondary to a faulty lumbar disc. A catheter is threaded into the disc tissue under fluoroscopic guidance. The catheter is composed of a thermal resistive coil (Figure 6.22). The coil is then heated, which leads to a modification of the fibers within the disc. Ultimately, the capsule of the disc becomes thicker, which may help to promote disc stability. In addition, IDET may cause destruction of nociceptors in the disc, thereby leading to reduction in pain. Few well-designed studies have been done regarding the short- and long-term efficacy of IDET, and treatment should be reserved for patients who have very well-documented low back pain that is the result of a degenerative or partially herniated disc.

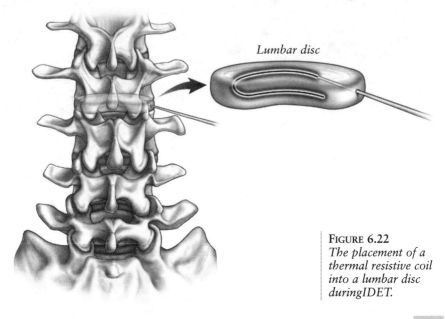

Lumbar disc

FIGURE 6.22
The placement of a thermal resistive coil into a lumbar disc duringIDET.

Summary Points

- Many nonsurgical options are available for patients who suffer with low back pain. Physical therapy or chiropractic treatment is usually the first line of treatment.
- Physical therapy should be provided by a therapist who specializes in treating lumbar spine conditions. The therapist should be willing to spend one-on-one time with the patient.
- Exercise is extremely valuable in managing low back pain. Meditative exercises can lead to a change in the body's physiology while helping to reduce pain.
- Acupuncture is often an effective treatment for acute low back pain, but should be integrated with other treatments when used for chronic pain.
- Therapeutic injections should be performed by a physician who has received specialized training. Other than trigger-point injections, therapeutic injections should be performed in an ambulatory surgery center or similar specialized center.

CHAPTER 7

Surgical Treatments

Spinal surgery may be an important aspect not only of pain management, but also in restoring neurologic or biomechanical stability. However, just as spinal surgery may ameliorate symptoms in patients with low back pain or related conditions, spinal surgery also may worsen symptoms. Some patients have multiple failed interventions, only to have another failed surgery in an attempt to rectify the pain. Two conditions necessitate performing immediate lumbar spine surgery:

- Loss of bowel control, bladder control, or both as a result of the lumbar spine condition.
- Rapidly progressive or absolute muscle weakness as a result of the low back condition.

A relative indication for low back surgery is that the patient has failed good, nonsurgical management for treatment of his low back condition, and the patient is presenting with a well-defined, anatomic basis as a cause of low back pain. As discussed earlier, it is more often the case that pain is driven by both anatomic and physiological factors. However, an astute clinician can discern when pain is primarily the result of an anatomic malfunction.

MEDICAL RISKS OF SURGERY

Before a patient can be considered for surgery, an internist or primary care physician and an anesthesiologist must assess the medical risks of surgery. Most lumbar spine surgery involves placing the patient under general anesthesia. This is a coma-like state in which the patient is *intubated*, which means that a ventilator is performing the action of breathing for the patient. While the patient is in this coma-like state, surgery can be performed painlessly, and the anesthesiologist monitors vital signs such as blood pressure and heartbeat.

General anesthesia and recovery from surgery place an extra stress on the heart. Therefore, the treating physicians must account for any possible weakness of the heart muscle or any possible blockage of the coronary arteries that supply blood to the heart muscle. Often, patients undergo special heart tests such as an exercise stress test and echocardiogram before they are cleared for surgery.

General anesthesia and recovery from surgery also stress the lungs. The lungs have a natural tendency to expand incompletely following surgery. In addition, because of pain following surgery, patients may be reluctant to take full, deep breaths. If the lungs do not expand fully with good deep breaths after surgery, then there is a risk of developing an infection or pneumonia following surgery. In patients who have compromised lung function to begin with—for example, chronic bronchitis or chronic obstructive pulmonary disease—then the risk of developing pneumonia or other lung problems increases, thus complicating surgery.

Some patients have other medical problems, such as diabetes and high blood pressure. General anesthesia and surgery can cause these medical conditions to worsen, especially following surgery, when the body is struggling to recover. Thus, all treating physicians must pay careful attention to monitoring and properly treating such conditions during and after surgery. Infection may develop following any surgery, and is more common in more complicated surgeries such as spinal fusion.

In essence, general anesthesia, surgery, and recovery from surgery place tremendous stress on the body in general, and the heart and lungs in particular. Younger, healthier patients generally have no difficulty tolerating such a procedure. However, medically ill or elderly patients deserve special consideration before they are cleared medically to undergo surgery, and they require intense monitoring following surgery.

LAMINECTOMY AND LAMINOTOMY

Laminectomy means that the lamina, which is part of the normally non-weight-bearing part of the lumbar spine, is partially cut so that the spinal surgeon (orthopedic surgeon or neurosurgeon) can view the contents of the spinal canal (Figure 7.1). Typically, just one side of the lamina is removed. However, if the surgeon requires more operating space, both sides of the lamina plus the posterior spinous process are removed (Figure 7.2). Following removal of part of the lamina, the surgeon can remove a fragment of a herniated disc or can perform techniques to widen the spinal canal, as is necessary in lumbar stenosis. (Lumbar stenosis, which is discussed in Chapter 13, is a degenerative condition of the spine that results in spinal canal narrowing.)

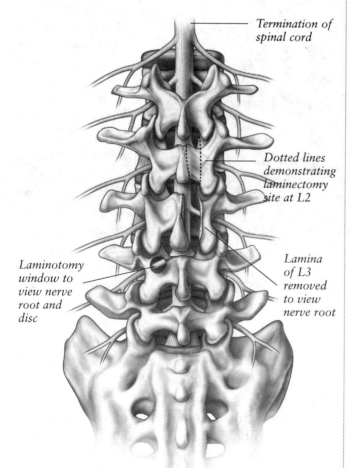

Termination of spinal cord

Dotted lines demonstrating laminectomy site at L2

Lamina of L3 removed to view nerve root

Laminotomy window to view nerve root and disc

FIGURE 7.1
The surgical approach for laminectomy and laminotomy.

101

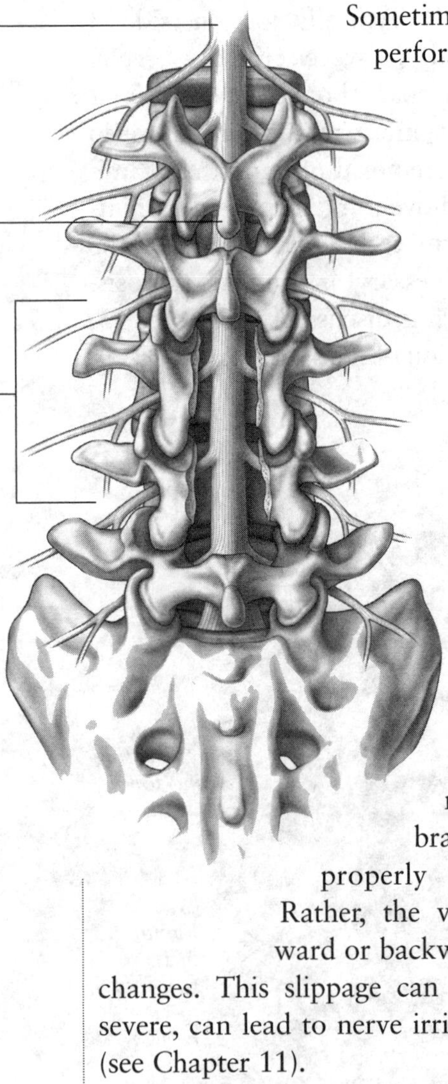

Termination of
spinal cord

Posterior
spinous process

Bilateral
laminectomy
at L3 and L4,
with removal
of lamina and
posterior
spinous
processes.

FIGURE 7.2
Multilevel
laminectomy.

Sometimes, a laminectomy is performed at more than one level (Figure 7.2). For example, a patient may present with two or more levels of disc herniation or lumbar stenosis that require surgery. Even though laminectomies can be performed at multiple levels, as the number of spinal joints affected increases, there is an increased risk for developing *spinal instability* following such surgery. Spinal instability means that the vertebrae no longer move in a properly coordinated manner. Rather, the vertebrae may slip forward or backward with body position changes. This slippage can cause pain and, when severe, can lead to nerve irritation or nerve damage (see Chapter 11).

Laminotomy means that a hole is drilled through part of the lamina. Laminotomies are performed when the surgeon requires only a small viewing area to perform surgery (Figure 7.1).

Recovery from laminectomy or laminotomy is generally within days. The patient may be discharged from the hospital within 1 or 2 days, and is walking immediately. Physical rehabilitation begins within a few weeks of the procedure. As with any surgical procedure, a risk of infection follows laminectomy or laminotomy, although the risk is small. Nerve damage is rare. The biggest risk is that the patient must undergo general anesthesia and must be medically fit to do so.

DISKECTOMY AND MICRODISKECTOMY

Diskectomy simply means that part of the lumbar disc is removed. Unless a spinal fusion procedure is performed, most diskectomies are done as part of a laminectomy or laminotomy. The purpose of the procedure is to remove that part of the disc that is placing pressure on a nerve or other pain-sensitive structure. The rest of the disc is left in place (Figure 7.3).

Microdiskectomy means that the entire surgical procedure is performed through a smaller incision, because the surgeon utilizes a microscope for the purpose of magnification. Diskectomy and microdiskectomy are appropriate procedures for herniated lumbar discs that are the primary anatomic basis of the patient's pain. An alternative to microdiskectomy is percutaneuos lumbar diskectomy, in which the surgery is performed through a small arthroscopic port; this procedure is less well-studied than microdiskectomy. The risks of diskectomy and microdiskectomy are similar to those of laminectomy.

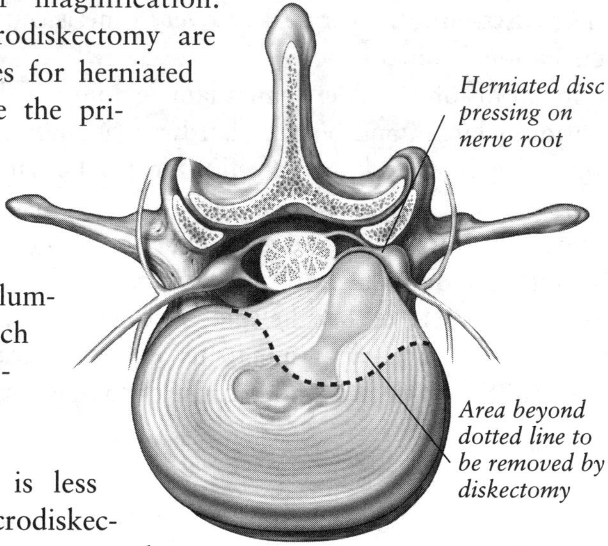

Herniated disc pressing on nerve root

Area beyond dotted line to be removed by diskectomy

FIGURE 7.3
Diskectomy.

103

SPINAL FUSION

Spinal fusion is performed when the spinal surgeon determines that the patient is at risk of developing spine instability. Spinal fusion can be done in several ways. Most commonly, the surgeon makes a large incision in the back, performs multilevel laminectomy, and then inserts metal rods and screws into the bony spine to assure stability (Figure 7.4).

In some cases, the surgeon will use a bone graft. A bone graft may come from a cadaver donor or may be from the patient's pelvis. A bone graft may be done in lieu of placing rods and screws, or it may be done in conjunction with the use of hardware.

In cases in which the surgeon feels the spine is at risk of becoming particularly unstable, spinal fusion surgery will be approached from both the back as well as abdominal region (circumferential fusion). This is a much more involved surgery, and the spinal surgeon usually works in conjunction with a general surgeon. The general surgeon performs the abdominal incision and layers the abdominal contents to the side so that the spinal surgeon has a good view of the spine once this is accomplished.

Some surgeons perform a minor incision, then place spinal fusion hardware using an arthroscopy-like instrument. This may be appropriate in select cases, and the surgical recovery time is much less than with more conventional spinal fusion.

Spinal fusion is riskier than a laminectomy or diskectomy. Because the incision is larger, and because hardware is inserted that is foreign to the body, a greater risk of infection from the large incision is present. Although recovery from a laminectomy is measured in days and weeks, recovery from spinal fusion takes at least 2 to 3 months. A patient is walking within 1 or 2 days, but must be rather cautious with movement in order to help assure that the spine fuses normally. A greater risk of nerve damage is possible with spinal fusion, both because of the larger-scale nature of the procedure and because of the placement of rods and screws near the nerves.

LUMBAR DISC REPLACEMENT

Lumbar disc replacement is becoming a new treatment option for some patients with back pain, specifically when the cause is degenerative disc

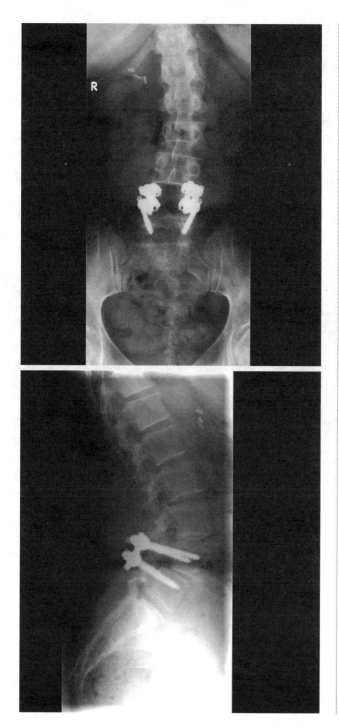

FIGURE 7.4
*Radiograph of a
patient with spinal
fusion hardware in
place.*

disease (see Chapter 11). The concept is similar to knee and hip replacement surgery in that the degenerative disc is replaced with a metal and plastic implant. The theoretical advantage of lumbar disc replacement surgery over spinal fusion is that some movement of the lumbar spine is restored with disc replacement, thus causing less stress on other spinal levels. Preliminary outcome studies are encouraging, but we do not have long-term data regarding effectiveness of treatment over time. In addition to the general risk of surgery, potential complications of disc replacement include vertebral body fracture, implant malposition, and difficulty with ejaculation in men. Some patients may additionally require spinal fusion despite lumbar disc replacement. In uncomplicated disc replacement surgery, recovery is generally within weeks.

REHABILITATION RISKS FOLLOWING SURGERY

Laminectomy and diskectomy procedures do not entail any significant risks with rehabilitation. The biggest risk is that some patients may feel quite well and attempt to return to their prior activity level prematurely. Generally speaking, patients should be limited to walking for the first month following laminectomy and diskectomy. Some spinal surgeons frown upon physical therapy, believing that the surgery alone is "curative." However, patients must realize that the herniated disc or other spinal condition that prompts surgery in the first place means that the spine is out of balance. After the patient is walking comfortably for 1 month following surgery, physical therapy with a therapist who specializes in spine stabilization helps to preserve long-term function and recovery of the low back.

Patients who undergo spinal fusion have more complicated rehabilitation needs. Although they are walking almost immediately, it is extremely important to ensure that the spinal fusion is successful. This means that any bone grafts must integrate completely into the bony spine and any hardware must become solidly fixed into the bony spine. Typically, the spinal surgeon will order serial radiographs of the spine to assess the progress of spine fusion (Figure 7.4). Full fusion may take 3 to 6 months.

During the first 3 to 6 months following spine fusion, patients are generally limited to walking as a form of exercise. Physical therapy and other exercises are discouraged because the spinal surgeon must be certain that no undue force is placed on the spine, thereby jeopardizing full integration of fusion. Once fusion is complete, many spinal surgeons simply ask patients to gradually increase activity as tolerated, but they do not recommend physical therapy. However, physical therapy with a focus on spine stabilization will help to assure that a new and healthy balance for the spine and its musculature develop, thus helping to assure long-term function and recovery of the low back.

RETURN TO FULL ACTIVITY

Most patients who undergo a simple laminectomy or diskectomy can return to full physical activity within months following surgery. The same may hold true for patients who have undergone successful lumbar disc replacement surgery, although long-term data are not available. Return to full activity assumes that the patient has achieved a renewed spine balance, ideally by working with a spine physical therapist and undergoing spine stabilization exercises. An exercise maintenance program helps to assure long-term, full recovery.

Patients who undergo spinal fusion may not be capable of returning to full physical activity, even if the fusion is completely successful. Once part of the spine is fused, greater stress is placed on the spinal joint above and below the fusion. Greater stress may also be placed on the hips. The increased stress develops as the body attempts to compensate for the lack of movement at the level of the spinal fusion. Thus, patients who are highly athletic or who perform heavy manual labor must modify their activities to avoid placing too much stress on the nonfused part of the spine.

Ideally, patients who undergo spinal fusion should work with a physical therapist who specializes in spine stabilization. Once patients understand the concepts of spine stabilization, they understand better what type of physical stress their body can safely withstand.

PAIN RISKS FOLLOWING SURGERY

Usually, spine surgery is performed to alleviate low back or leg pain from the spinal condition for which it is recommended. In patients who have chronic pain prior to surgery, a much greater risk is present of an increase in chronic pain following surgery. This is a much-overlooked aspect of spine surgery risk. Too often, the patient is assessed simply from an anatomic and medical viewpoint, but the true nature of the pain is not completely understood.

Those patients who have straightforward pain that correlates well with the level of the spine for which surgery is recommended are more likely to develop pain relief following surgery. Prior to surgery, these patients generally can become comfortable in certain positions (for example, lying down), and develop pain in other positions (for example, walking). In addition, these patients have pain that has persisted for months, as opposed to years.

On the other hand, some patients present with chronic pain of many months' or years' duration, and the pain is seemingly independent of any activity. The patient may be diagnosed with a degenerative or herniated lumbar disc, and he may be offered the hope that corrective surgery will alleviate pain. However, herniated and degenerative lumbar discs should not cause chronic, essentially constant pain. Patients with chronic pain require intense nonsurgical treatment with a pain medicine specialist or within a pain center. Surgery for such patients usually is not only disappointing, but may lead to a marked worsening of preoperative pain.

SPINAL CORD STIMULATION

Spinal cord stimulation is based on the *gate theory* of pain. In this theory, stimulation of one part of the nervous system can override the pain pathways; thus, the patient's perception of pain is lessened or becomes minimal. Spinal cord stimulation is achieved by placement of a spinal cord stimulator, which is somewhat similar to a heart pacemaker. Electrodes are placed in the epidural space, which is the same space utilized for epidural injections. The electrodes are connected to an internalized pulse generator and, if the initial screening is favorable, then the generator is placed internally, usually within the abdominal cavity (Figure 7.5). This generator can be modified by use of an external magnet.

Spinal cord stimulator placement should be performed only in patients who have well-localized pain and who have received other aspects of multidisciplinary pain management. Spinal cord stimulation is not used for treatment of acute pain. Rather, spinal cord stimulation is a strategy that is chosen for patients with chronic, neuropathic pain conditions. Such

conditions can include well-localized low back pain or well-localized radiating leg pain.

Even under the best of circumstances, the success rate for spinal
cord stimulation is only about 50%.
This procedure should not be used as
part of a rapid escalation of intervention in patients with chronic pain.
It is best utilized in patients who
have received a combination of
physical therapy, pharmacologic management, and psychotherapy, and who have a
firm commitment to ongoing
self-care.

A risk of infection is possible with the placement of a

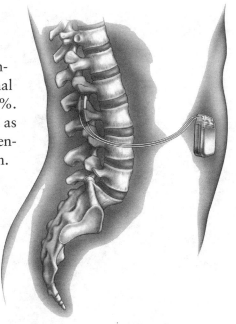

FIGURE 7.5
Spinal cord stimulator.

spinal cord stimulator and, when this occurs, the
device usually must be removed. The wires within
the epidural space can migrate, making the stimulation ineffective and necessitating further surgery.
Some patients do not like the feel of the generator,
which is placed in the abdominal region. The generator can fail, necessitating further surgery for
replacement.

MORPHINE PUMP

As discussed in Chapter 5, narcotic analgesics are
the most potent analgesics available for the treatment of pain. Some patients who suffer with chronic pain cannot tolerate the systemic side effects of
oral narcotics. Such side effects may include severe
constipation, lethargy, or both. For patients who
have participated in multidisciplinary pain management and who respond beneficially to narcotics but

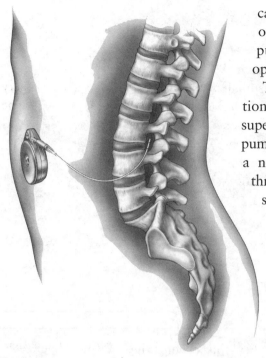

FIGURE 7.6
Morphine pump.

cannot tolerate large doses of oral narcotics, a morphine pump may be a reasonable option.

The pump, containing medication in its reservoir, is placed superficially in the abdomen. The pump is refilled periodically using a needle to access the reservoir through a small opening in the skin. The pump is attached to a catheter that is placed within the lumbar spinal canal (Figure 7.6). The pump is programmed to deliver medication at a rate determined by the clinician and the patient, depending on the patient's pain patterns and needs.

Morphine pump treatment takes advantage of the fact that narcotic (opiate) receptors are located in the spine and, if these receptors are activated, a much smaller dose of medication can be used (about one-one-hundredth of the oral dose). Thus, the systemic side effects are minimized. Although morphine pumps initially were used for patients suffering with cancer pain, they are now an acceptable treatment alternative for some patients with chronic low back or neuropathic pain.

A risk of infection is possible with morphine pump placement. Sometimes the catheter that delivers the medicine will kink or close because of scar tissue, necessitating further surgery. Some patients do not like the feel of the morphine pump, which is usually placed in the abdomen.

SUMMARY POINTS

- Spine surgery is but one avenue that may be appropriate in patients who have low back conditions.

- Two absolute indications that necessitate immediate spine surgery include (a) loss of bowel or bladder control as a result of the spine condition and (b) rapidly progressive or absolute muscle weakness as a result of the spine condition.

- The type of surgery performed is based on the surgeon's assessment of the cause of pain, as well as the stability of the spine.

- Spine surgery is not a cure for patients with nonspecific, chronic low back pain. For patients who suffer with chronic pain, spine surgery may cause a worsening of pain symptoms.

- The medical risks of surgery must be considered carefully by all treating physicians. Sometimes, the medical and rehabilitation risks of surgery outweigh the possible benefit of performing surgery.

- Spinal cord stimulation may help some patients with well-localized neuropathic pain in the low back or leg. A morphine pump may help some patients who require and benefit from narcotic analgesics, but who cannot tolerate their side effects when take orally.

CHAPTER 8

Mind–Body and Integrative Strategies

MIND–BODY

Mind–body refers to the practice of understanding the relationship between thought and emotions on the one hand, and the physical body on the other. Philosophers and theologians have debated the origin and essence of thought for years. From a neuroscience perspective, thought is the result of brain processes, and thought is perceived within the human body as a result of the activation of physical pathways.

Emotions, Chemicals, and Receptors

Fear is associated with muscle contraction, pupil dilation, and a heightened state of awareness. Love is associated with muscle relaxation, giddy behavior, and an increased sense of well-being. Rage is associated with piloerection (arm hairs standing on end), forceful heart muscle contractility, and a diminution of rational feedback on action.

Functional brain imaging studies demonstrate that certain thought patterns are associated with metabolic or physiologic changes within certain areas of the brain. In addition, neuroscience and immunologic studies have revealed a key link between the emotions and related receptors throughout the body.

As discussed in Chapter 5, the body has an innate narcotic or opiate system, which means that the body produces its own morphine-like chemicals. These chemicals are released into the body and make connections with specific receptors. A chemical–receptor connection works in a manner similar to a lock and key. When the chemical connects with a receptor that matches its properties, a specified chemical–physical reaction occurs. When the mind–body is in a relaxed, peaceful, or euphoric

112

state, the innate opiate receptors are activated by the body's own release of opiates.

With the body's opiates, the reaction can range from pain control to an enhanced immune response, depending on the location of the reaction. For example, the white blood cell, whose normal purpose is to provide immune balance and to fight infection, contains opiate receptors. When the opiate receptor on the white blood cell is primed (a connection is made with the opiate chemical), the white blood cell functions better than when it is not primed. This could mean that, under situations of distress, white blood cell function is less effective, and a person may be more prone to infection. Thus, in this complex scenario, prolonged distress may make one more vulnerable to infection because of the manner in which the emotions manifest in the body.

The spinal cord contains numerous opiate receptors. When the body produces adequate opiates internally, this helps control pain that otherwise might be expressed. Morphine-like medications can take advantage of an inability to produce adequate opiates internally, because they also bind to receptors to help control pain.

Serotonin is a neurochemical that is simplistically thought of as the "happy" neurochemical. The new-generation antidepressant medications work primarily by making serotonin more available to the brain. Because serotonin plays a key role in promoting a sense of well-being, such medications are useful adjuncts in the treatment of depression. The inadequate production of serotonin may be associated with anxiety or depression. Interestingly, the intestines have innumerable serotonin receptors. When the body's serotonin production is dysfunctional, intestinal irritability may develop.

EMOTIONAL PROCESSING AND CHRONIC PAIN

If we analyze in more detail the pathways involved in mediating chronic pain, we come to understand that many areas of the brain that are normally involved in nonconscious and emotional processing are intimately linked to mediating the perception of chronic pain. For example, scientific studies have demonstrated a remarkable similarity in many brain pathways when we compare patients with neuropathic pain with post-traumatic stress disorder patients. This does not mean that patients with post-traumatic stress disorder have neuropathic pain or that patients with neuropathic pain have post-traumatic stress disorder. Rather, this means that both groups of patients have dysfunctional brain pathways, and these pathways lead to either the pain state or the heightened anxiety state.

What is not so well understood at present is why certain brain pathways that normally function for emotional processing become activated in chronic pain. We simply know that this is the case. We can combine this scientific knowledge with other clinical studies that have demonstrated an increase in chronic pain among individuals who have suffered considerable prior physical or emotional upheaval. We must be cautious in interpreting these studies, because they do not imply that all people who have suffered considerable upheaval will develop pain, or that patients with chronic pain have been victims of some physical or emotional abuse. Rather, we can say that, in some cases, chronic pain is associated with prior, significant physical and emotional distress, and that the brain pathways that are linked to this distress can begin to manifest in turning on certain pain circuits.

As we often dissociate from our emotions, this link between the emotional brain and the pain pathways may make sense. This may be the body's way of calling attention to itself, in essence trying to give a message that something is wrong. Because of our physical bias, we always consider first that the "something wrong" must be an anatomic lesion. Because we now understand that chronic pain is very often mediated by a physiologic perturbation or dysfunction in the nervous system, we need to consider further that such dysfunction may have manifestations in our thought processes and emotions as well as in our anatomic structures. Sometimes, the dysfunction arises because of an inciting event that may be linked to another emotionally charged and unresolved reality within oneself.

It might be easier to understand the principle of mind–body and integrative medicine through the following examples.

Example 1

A 50-year-old male patient presented to the office with complaints of severe low back pain. He recalls that 3 days earlier, he was taking out the garbage, and he developed a sudden twinge of pain in his lower back. Within hours, he was pitched forward and had difficulty standing straight. He became essentially bed-bound with incapacitating pain and sought advice about his condition.

The patient's examination was notable for a reproduction of pain with forward trunk flexion or with raising his legs while his knees were in an extended position. He had no neurologic abnormalities. He walked with a limp because of pain.

Ultimately, the patient was diagnosed with a herniated lumbar disc. At a simplistic level, the patient developed a lumbar disc herniation because he was carrying heavy garbage, the biomechanical load was more than his spine could handle, and this led to an annular tear and subsequent herniation of a lumbar disc. This story could end here and treatment could be directed at helping the patient control his pain, then recommending a course of physical therapy.

What generally is not addressed in such a scenario is the patient's state of being at the time he was taking out the garbage. In this particular case, the patient was in a state of considerable distress, because he was fearful of losing his job. In addition, marital discord was present, in large part because of disagreement as how to best raise their troubled teenage son. On the particular night in which the patient developed low back pain, it was raining outside, the patient's wife was nagging him to take out the garbage, and the patient's teenage son was in the basement, oblivious to everything except TV. It was in this setting that the patient developed the herniated lumbar disc.

When the mind–body is in a state of considerable distress, the muscles may contract abnormally, possibly without our conscious realization. In addition, under heightened stress and anxiety, certain emotional pathways that cross-link with pain can become activated. In this particular patient, he likely had considerable abnormal muscle contraction around the lumbar spine, and this may have led to such imbalance that his lumbar disc could no longer support what his body was trying to do.

We need not look into this too deeply and conclude that every case of a lumbar disc herniation is associated with a complex psychosocial history. However, it is exceedingly useful to consider the patient's deeper perception at the time of an inciting event. Specifically, rather than simply looking for a concrete physical cause of a sudden pain syndrome, we may step back and try to understand the entire event or chain of events that ultimately led to the low back pain syndrome. If this does reveal a source of psychosocial distress, then treatment is not simply directed at the anatomic basis of pain, but also is directed at helping the patient to make healthy lifestyle changes.

In this patient, his management was multidisciplinary. He was treated initially with an oral corticosteroid and narcotic analgesic. Once he obtained pain relief from the medication, he began physical therapy and also agreed to begin stress management classes. The patient recovered completely, and he has done well over the long term.

Example 2

A 45-year-old female presented to the office with complaints of intractable low back pain. She recalls having had a history of low back pain as a child. She is somewhat vague about the details, but states that ultimately this back pain cleared, and she was rather athletic in her teenage years, playing intramural sports while she attended college. She had been pregnant three times, suffered one miscarriage and had two uneventful deliveries otherwise, and did not suffer with back pain during pregnancy.

Her current pain began about 5 years ago. She notes that she fell downstairs, did not lose consciousness, and did not have sudden, severe pain after falling down the stairs. However, during the next several days, she developed increasing symptoms of low back pain without radiating pain into the buttock or leg region. She sought treatment with a chiropractor and, despite adjustments three times weekly over a period of 1 year, she did not improve. She then sought treatment with an orthopedic surgeon, who recommended nonsteroidal anti-inflammatory drugs and physical therapy. Again, this treatment led to no substantial pain relief.

The patient underwent a series of diagnostic tests. Plain radiographs of the lumbar spine were essentially normal. MRI of the lumbar spine revealed two-level degenerative disc changes, without a significant herniated lumbar disc, and with some associated facet degenerative changes. Rheumatologic blood work-up was negative. She was evaluated by a pain anesthesiologist, and he treated her with a series of lumbar facet injections, which provided minimal, if any, pain relief. The pain anesthesiologist then recommended a rhizotomy procedure, which yielded no positive benefit. She then underwent a series of lumbar epidural corticosteroid injections and obtained no pain relief. The pain anesthesiologist then told the patient that she was a candidate for a spinal cord stimulator, and the spinal cord stimulator trial was unsuccessful.

The patient then saw a spine surgeon, who recommended lumbar spine fusion. At the time of evaluation, the patient had pain that was across the entire area of the low back. The pain was essentially constant. It sometimes had a burning quality to it; otherwise, she described it as a deep, aching pain. The pain seemed at its worst when she was lying supine, and pain could awaken the patient from her sleep. She did not have excruciating pain on first standing in the morning. The pain persisted during the day, but as she was increasingly physically active, she seemed to be less aware of the pain. She did walk about 1 mile daily and, although she was not free of pain while walking, the pain did not worsen with walking. She otherwise was feeling well and in good health, maintaining a stable weight pattern and menstruating regularly while being free of fevers, chills, and sweats.

The spine surgeon explained to the patient that she should undergo lumbar spine fusion because of the persistence of her pain, the failure of all conservative management, and the two-level abnormality noted on the lumbar spine MRI study. He performed spinal fusion surgery.

Although the surgery was uncomplicated from a technical and medical point of view, she developed increasingly severe pain following the surgery. This pain persisted for a period of 2 years and only worsened with time. The basic characteristics of the pain remained the same, other than that the intensity, especially at night, was worse.

She then began a new course of treatment in a multidisciplinary pain center. It was noted that she was considerably depressed. She felt that she could not participate meaningfully in the care of her children. She had discontinued working because of pain. She was estranged from her husband but not formally divorced. She increasingly withdrew from her social contacts, and her only meaningful outside activity was her daily walk.

She had no panic or anxiety attacks, although she stated that she had a previous history of a panic disorder that had resolved over time. She essentially felt hopeless, believing that she would never be free of pain, and that there was nothing that anyone could offer to her.

Her management consisted of working with a psychologist, a physical therapist, a massage therapist who was trained in working with chronic pain patients, and a neurologist who coordinated her medical care and prescribed medication. Her medication included a combination of an anti-depressant medication, an anticonvulsant medication, and a narcotic analgesic. She understood that she was receiving an antidepressant medication to help stabilize her mood and to help with some aspects of pain control. She understood that the anticonvulsant medication was to help to relieve pain. Although she was fearful of taking a narcotic, she agreed to use this medication judiciously, and she signed a contract indicating the parameters under which she could take this medication.

With the psychologist, the sessions focused primarily on her maladaptive psychosocial situation. She began to open up more and more, to discuss her frustration and to discuss some of the difficulties with her estranged husband. The psychologist had a sense that other aspects of her history might be more revealing, but did not press the patient, understanding that if other significant aspects of her psychological history were present, they must be volunteered from the patient, and not suggested from the psychologist.

The physical therapy treatment focused initially on craniosacral technique. In this setting, the patient would lie quietly on a table as the therapist worked intuitively from the sacrum to the head region, encouraging the patient to become more meditative and to learn to work with her body as the therapist was performing this technique. Initially, the patient was extraordinarily frightened even to lie supine, and she preferred to undergo treatment from a seated position. On two occasions, the patient began sobbing inconsolably while undergoing therapy, but wished not to discuss her emotions or perceptions further.

The patient also underwent group therapy treatment, which consists of a skilled group leader working with six patients who suffer with chronic pain. During the group therapy sessions, participants practiced several behavioral tools, including meditative and relaxation techniques, and they came to understand the concept of turning inward as opposed to simply focusing on physical pain.

Over time, the patient made small gains, and she developed a sense of trust with her health care practitioners. During one group therapy session, the patient began to cry and shared considerable details about her past history. This included a history of having been gang raped as a child. During this experience, she was held and kicked repeatedly in the lower back region. It was following this episode that the patient developed low back pain during her earlier years, and she underwent psychotherapy to help her cope with the rape. In the patient's mind, she had compartmentalized this event, had moved beyond it, and did not think that it was relevant any longer.

The patient recounted further that the events leading to her current bout of back pain began with a fight with her alcoholic husband. During a physical altercation, she was kicked down the stairs. Out of fear, she never reported this event, but she did find the courage to separate herself from this abusive relationship.

The separated husband controlled the patient's finances, and he used this control to punish both the patient and their two teenage children. The patient felt trapped, with no recourse for action. It was within this setting—this conceptual framework—that the patient had undergone multiple treatments for her chronic back pain. Nobody had taken a careful social or psychological history and, because the patient was suffering with physical pain, she did not think that her personal upheaval was linked to her physical low back pain.

With increasing group and personal psychological counseling, the patient came to trust her treating clinicians, and more important, she began to trust herself. One profoundly insightful session led to the realization that she always blamed herself for having been raped as a child. Deep down, she felt that she was somehow worthless and forever stained, and that she deserved the abuse she received. Her rational mind stated otherwise, but her basic sense of self was always kindling guilt, shame, and a sense of worthlessness.

On realizing that she suffered from a profound lack of self-esteem, the patient also came to realize that the events in her marriage were similarly commingled with poor self-esteem and self-blame. Ultimately, the patient allowed herself to relive the perceptions of herself when she was pushed down the stairs by her alcoholic husband. This event previously had awakened a profound sense of shame, guilt, and self-loathing, and this realization was unacceptable to her rational mind. In dissociating from this realization, her physical pain became the primary expression of her deep-seated emotional pain.

The patient struggled with her perception of guilt and self-loathing, but with persistent positive feedback and intense group and one-on-one psychotherapy, she transformed this perception into one of self-care and self-love. This is no easy task. Even when we believe rationally that we should love ourselves, the body responds to the core belief of self-perception rather than the mask of rationalization.

Over a period of 2 years, the patient became more engaged in a new social life, and she dedicated herself to intense self-care. She has become essentially pain free, is working full-time, and feels very connected to her two children. She also has become a group leader for abused and battered women.

INTERPRETING MIND–BODY EXAMPLES

These examples demonstrate the enormous complexity of mind–body work. Since the age of Descartes, who championed the notion of the superiority of the rational mind, our Western culture has equated rational thinking with the mind, yet neuroscience and other clinical work tell us otherwise. We know, for example, from eloquent experiments in patients who have undergone surgery to remove the connection between the left hemisphere and right hemisphere of the brain, that the left hemisphere will fabricate an explanation for behavior generated from the right hemisphere. Normally, the left hemisphere of the brain is responsible for our rational way of interpreting life or for rationalizing why we behave as we do. The right hemisphere is more dedicated to our creative and emotional intelligence. In some patients with severe epilepsy, the connection between the two hemispheres is surgically removed, thus preventing a spread of epilepsy from one side of the brain to another. These patients are known as *split-brain patients*.

In the eloquent experiments conducted on split-brain patients, a command can be given, through sophisticated visual cues, to either the right or left hemisphere. If the right hemisphere is given a command to follow, such as waving the left hand, the split-brain patient will wave the hand but the left side of the brain does not know why. Then, the left brain can be asked why "he" is waving, and the left brain will fabricate (rationalize) an explanation, completely believing the validity of the false rationalization.

In addition to the split-brain experiments, we know from the writings of William James (an American psychologist who described the unconscious mind before Freud) and from functional brain imaging studies, that the physiologic and physical expressions of emotions such as fear precede conscious awareness of fear. Thus, the startle response—pupil dilation, muscle contraction, piloerection, and hypervigilance—occurs almost instantaneously following a sudden threatening environmental cue, all before the individual becomes aware that he is even afraid. In other words, the body generates an emotional response before the individual is consciously aware of the emotion. The rational mind does not determine the emotion; rather, the rational mind may choose to clarify, modify, or compartmentalize the emotion. The rational mind may even choose to ignore the emotion.

These clinical examples must be considered within a conceptual frame-work of two key scientific discoveries: (a) emotional circuits in the brain often are dysfunctional in chronic pain patients, and these circuits maintain the perception of pain; and (b) the rational brain will provide an explanation for events that may have nothing to do with reality and that may serve to protect the individual from a reality from which the person is more comfortable ignoring or compartmentalizing. In the second example, it was only after the patient came to truly "walk through" and accept her deepest emotional truth that she was able to begin to transform her chronic pain.

Our true understanding of the implications of the emotional brain is in its infancy, especially as it pertains to chronic pain. Any understanding, with clinical implications, must be rooted in science and must be free of judgment. In this second example, the patient came to understand that she could express herself and explore her perceptions without fear of judgment. Ultimately, her clinical improvement occurred not simply because of her realizations, but because she felt she could safely explore her life—her interpretation of life—in a clinical setting that was free of judgment and full of clinical support and human compassion.

SUMMARY POINTS

- Mind–body refers to the interplay between thought and emotions with the body.
- Emotional pathways often are interlinked with chronic pain pathways.
- Emotions often are expressed physiologically and physically before there is a conscious awareness of the emotion.

- The left hemisphere of the brain is primarily responsible for rational thought, but may also be responsible for rationalizing an interpretation of reality, even if that interpretation is not grounded in truth.
- We must be cautious in mind–body medicine not to form premature judgments about a possible emotional cause of pain.

Low Back Pain Syndromes

CHAPTER 9

Lumbar Strain

CLINICAL PRESENTATION

Acute lumbar strain is probably the most common cause of low back pain. Unfortunately, this is also commonly misdiagnosed when patients first present with low back pain. By definition, acute lumbar strain should be a short-lived, self-limited cause of low back pain. Typically, patients present with a rather sudden onset of pain that is localized to one side of the lower back or sometimes diffusely across the lower back. Pain may radiate into the buttock region and rarely into the leg, but usually the pain is localized to the lower back.

Most patients develop lumbar strain as part of an overuse pattern. That is, either the patient has repetitively engaged in an activity for which the lumbar spine is inadequately prepared, or the patient has engaged in a more sudden strenuous activity that overloads the normal muscular support structure of the lumbar spine. Typically, patients are comfortable lying down or sitting and feel increased pain when standing or, especially, with certain bending motions of the spine. Otherwise, patients are medically well.

CAUSE OF LUMBAR STRAIN

Although the exact cause of lumbar strain is not completely clear-cut, a pattern generally occurs in which supporting musculature of the lumbar spine is relatively underdeveloped relative to the demands placed on it. This leads to a situation of muscle fatigue that increases vulnerability for a sudden stretch or tear of the muscle, possibly with associated spasm.

PHYSICAL EXAMINATION

The physical examination is largely unremarkable. A palpable area of muscle spasm may be present if the muscle group involved is the erector spinae. Pain may be reproduced with resistance to back extension or lateral movement. The neurologic examination is normal.

IMAGING AND DIAGNOSTIC STUDIES

Imaging and diagnostic studies are not required for acute lumbar strain. The clinical presentation is straightforward, and because the imaging studies are unrevealing, they should be performed only if there is doubt as to the diagnosis or if symptoms persist. A plain radiograph may reveal evidence of muscle spasm by way of straightening of the normal curvature of the spine.

TREATMENT CONSIDERATIONS

Nonsurgical

Most patients can be managed with a simple regimen, and should be able to return to full activity within days, or at most, within weeks. Local application of ice may be helpful if an area of muscle spasm is present, and ice application usually provides immediate pain relief.

For the patient who has more severe pain, the medication of choice is a muscle relaxant. This helps to alleviate symptoms, and it allows the patient to resume physical activities without discomfort. Nonsteroidal anti-inflammatory drugs (NSAIDs) are less beneficial for acute lumbar strain. Although they are almost provided as a reflex when patients see a physician, they are not necessary because no significant degree of inflammation occurs in acute lumbar strain. Similarly, corticosteroids should not be prescribed. Narcotic analgesics should only be used for patients with quite severe lumbar strain.

Hands-on treatment is quite helpful in lumbar strain. Spinal manipulation is usually efficacious in alleviating symptoms of lumbar strain. Physical therapy is useful if the focus is on a myofascial release and other manual techniques. Acupuncture can lead to a regional myofascial release that, in association with *chi* balancing, can alleviate symptoms.

Once the patient has achieved reasonable pain relief, a concerted effort should be made to understand the muscle imbalance that led to lumbar strain. Often, the muscle imbalance is coupled with a psychological or psychosocial imbalance and, ideally, both should be addressed.

Surgical

There are no indications for surgical interventions in lumbar strain.

MIND–BODY CONSIDERATIONS

Although lumbar strain may simply be the result of a "weekend warrior" mentality, there are important mind–body considerations. Very often, patients are engaged in activity in which they are overextending themselves, both physically and psychologically. Some patients simply are neglecting the demands they are placing on their bodies because of a desire to perform, excel, or succeed, relative to some preordained value scale. In some cases, lumbar strain may occur in the setting of job dissatisfaction and repeated activities in which the patient is out of balance, both physically and emotionally. Even though lumbar strain may be a self-limited phenomenon, it is useful to guide patients so that they can gain insight into what leads to lumbar strain. In situations of undue anxiety or stress, some patients may be predisposed to abnormal contractures of the lumbar spinal musculature, and repetitive workloads in the setting of such abnormal contractures also predispose to lumbar strain.

Relaxation and meditative strategies in conjunction with hands-on therapy as described in the section on Nonsurgical Treatment lead to a successful healing in the vast majority of cases of lumbar strain.

ILLUSTRATIVE CASE

A 20-year-old male tennis player presented with the sudden onset of low back pain. Although he is a professional tennis player, he never qualified for a Grand Slam tournament and, at the time of presentation, he had his best opportunity to gain entry into the main draw of the U.S. Open Tennis Championships. For 1 week, he had endured a grueling hard court schedule, and he was currently playing the qualifying tournament for the U.S. Open Tennis Championships.

For the weeks prior to presentation, the player was essentially competing without adequate rest between matches, and he was doing no training otherwise. He felt considerable pressure from his overbearing father and from his exceedingly nervous coach. He had a sense that if he did not succeed in gaining entry into this U.S. Open Tennis Championships, he would need to seek another career.

On the day of presentation, the patient was in the second set of a match. He developed the sudden onset of pain in the left lower back while attempting to serve. The pain was sufficiently severe that he was unable to continue playing, and he retired from the match. He was initially quite distraught when evaluated, and this was compounded by the fact that his father was demanding a simple fix to the problem. Once the father left the examination room, the patient began to cry. He revealed the considerable stress and pressure he felt internally.

The physical exam was fairly unremarkable, although the patient demonstrated pivotal sacro-iliac movement with trunk extension and flexion, which suggests deep rotator muscle imbalance. His neurological exam was normal, and he was diagnosed with probable multifidus muscle lumbar strain.

Ultimately, it became clear that the patient's training regimen was wholly inadequate for the demands being placed on him. It was also clear that he had little downtime for self-reflection or for even listening to what his body was trying to tell him. He had been exhausted for weeks, but kept pushing himself, always with the single-minded goal of gaining entry into the U.S. Open Tennis Championships.

The patient agreed to take 1 month off from tennis and to use this time to work with a physical therapist and begin some self-reflection. This included meditative breathing exercises. He was given a muscle relaxant for short-term management of pain.

The physical therapy program focused on assessing his muscle imbalance. It was noted that his deep lumbar rotator muscles, as well as his extensor back muscles, were quite weak compared to his abdominal muscles. He began a program with progressive spine stabilization, became more self-confident and self-aware, and returned to successful tennis playing. He has remained asymptomatic.

Author's Note

This case demonstrates a clear mind–body continuum in a young athlete struggling to succeed. This case is not too different from anyone else who is struggling to succeed but is taking little time for self-reflection and proper exercise, especially to assure fitness for the demands being placed upon the body. Generally speaking, when patients present with lumbar strain, one can discern that both the mind and the body have reached a place of imbalance. Once this is recognized, successful management is relatively easy.

SUMMARY POINTS

- Lumbar strain is the most common cause of low back pain; it is usually short-lived and self-limited.
- Most patients develop lumbar strain because of physical imbalance, emotional imbalance, or both.
- Muscle relaxants, acupuncture, spinal manipulation, and hands-on physical therapy are effective treatments for lumbar strain.
- Patients with lumbar strain should try to reflect on how they developed a mind-body imbalance.

CHAPTER 10

Lumbar Disc Herniation

CLINICAL PRESENTATION

As discussed in Chapter 2, the lumbar disc is comprised of an inner gel and an outer annulus. The lumbar discs provide stability and resiliency to the lumbar spine. Lumbar disc herniation develops because of a tear in the annulus of the lumbar spine; the inner nucleus pulposus extends beyond the tear, compromising a part of the spinal canal (Figure 10.1). In many cases, lumbar disc herniation develops insidiously as a result of repeated, small micro tears that develop in conjunction with a degenerative disc. In these cases, patients with lumbar disc herniation may be completely without symptoms. Indeed, modern

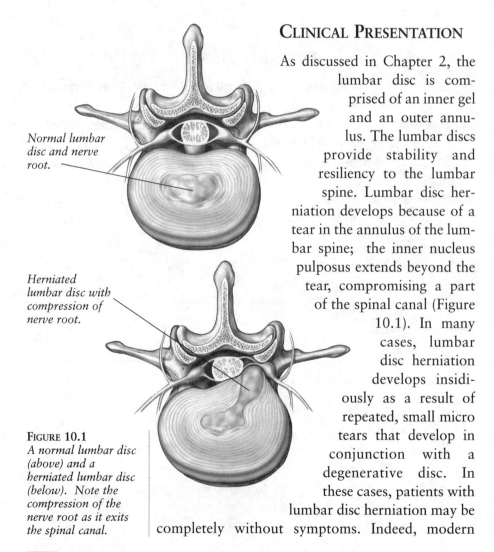

Normal lumbar disc and nerve root.

Herniated lumbar disc with compression of nerve root.

FIGURE 10.1
A normal lumbar disc (above) and a herniated lumbar disc (below). Note the compression of the nerve root as it exits the spinal canal.

imaging studies have revealed that lumbar disc herniations may be present in a sizable number of individuals who have no symptoms.

Many patients with an acute lumbar disc herniations have symptoms of pain or numbness in conjunction with a pinched or compressed nerve. Acute lumber disc herniation develops because of a sudden and large tear in the annulus, with subsequent rupture of nucleus pulposus material through the tear. Most of these herniations occur posteriorly, that is, toward the back. They also are generally to one side, but occasionally are midline.

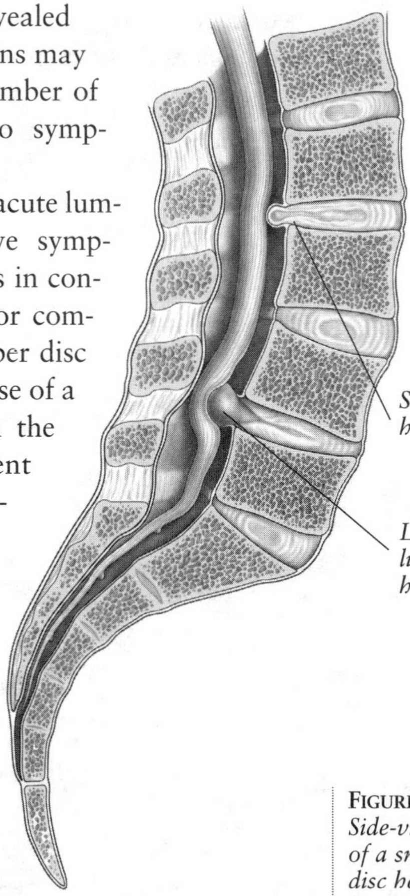

If a disc herniation is initially midline, pain is perceived as a deep discomfort in the center of the lower back. Sometimes patients describe a sudden popping sensation. Other times, the patient senses that something is wrong in the lower back, but the pain may not be excruciating. Over days, the tear may enlarge and the disc herniation worsens while symptoms increase (Figure 10.2).

As a disc herniation enlarges, it generally does so to the right or left of midline. Often, it will compress the lumbar nerve root at that level. Most disc herniations develop between L4–L5, or L5–S1, which are the two lowest segments of the lumbar spine. These

Small lumbar disc herniation

Large acute lumbar disc herniation

FIGURE 10.2
Side-view illustration of a small lumbar disc herniation and a large lumbar disc herniation. Note that the small herniation causes minimal pressure on the spinal canal.

two levels of the lumbar spine are the most mobile and vulnerable segments (Figure 10.3).

When a nerve root is compressed, there may be associated pain, and pain will normally be perceived

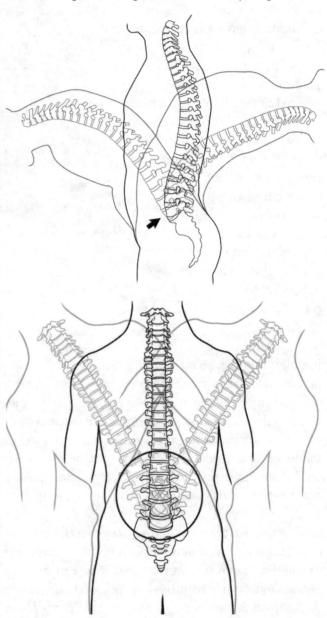

Figure 10.3
Spinal mobility in the lumbar spine, with most mobility occurring in the low lumbar spine.

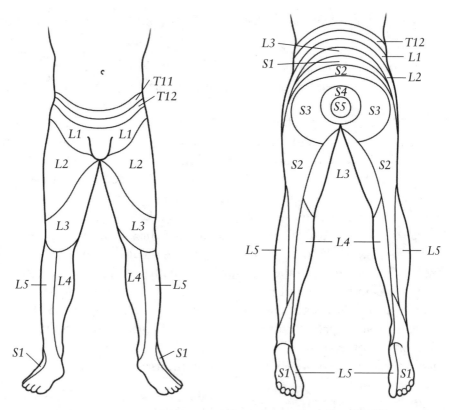

FIGURE 10.4
The sensory distribution of the nerves.

in the sensory distribution of that nerve (Figure 10.4). For example, a herniated disc at L4-5 may compress either the right or left L5 nerve root, which may cause pain radiating down the right or left side of the leg and into the great toe. If the nerve is severely compressed, there may be numbness (corresponding to the same sensory distribution) or muscle weakness. This demands urgent neurological evaluation.

Patients with acute lumbar disc herniation typically are comfortable lying on their back with knees flexed. Sitting is often uncomfortable, and standing may or may not be comfortable. Patients generally avoid bending forward, and sudden coughing or sneezing can worsen symptoms.

CAUSE OF LUMBAR DISC HERNIATION

The cause of acute lumbar disc herniation is not always apparent. Patients with chronic, degenerative lumbar discs and associated disc herniations often have a genetic predisposition to such degenerative changes. Otherwise, lumbar disc herniations generally occur in the setting of repeated overuse of the lumbar spine or sudden, more severe overuse. In this case, it is not simply the supporting musculature that gives, but the stabilizing force of the lumbar spine itself.

For degenerative lumbar disc herniations, the inner contents of the nucleus pulposus undergo a gradual change, which leads to a loss of water content in the nucleus pulposus. This drier disc makes the annulus susceptible to repeated micro tears. For an acute annular disc tear, the inner nucleus pulposus is generally healthy, and the water content is normal or near normal. The ultimate clinical expression of a lumbar disc herniation depends on the size and location of the disc. Large, midline central disc herniations cause primarily low back pain and, if they are severe, may lead to a worrisome neurologic presentation (discussed next). Discs that lateralize to one side or the other generally are associated with radiating leg symptoms, appropriate to the nerve root that is compromised (see Figure 10.4).

PHYSICAL EXAMINATION

Patients with acute lumbar disc herniation are generally in considerable pain. They may be tilted to one side or the other, especially if the nerve root is compromised (Figure 10.5). Forward bending generally is quite uncomfortable. From a seated position, a straight leg-raising maneuver, as demonstrated in Figure 10.6, may reproduce the patient's pain by stretching the compressed nerve. Areas of palpable muscle spasm may be present in the lower back. Even if a nerve root is compromised, the neurologic exam may be normal. If nerve compression is severe enough, then there may be a loss of sensation, a loss of reflex, or motor weakness that corresponds to the level of nerve dysfunction.

IMAGING AND DIAGNOSTIC STUDIES

Although plain radiographs are often obtained in the work-up of patients with lumbar disc herniation, they are generally unhelpful. The usefulness of a plain radiograph is more for excluding other causes of back and radiating leg pain. Magnetic resonance imaging (MRI) is the diagnostic study of choice for lumbar disc herniation. If the clinician suspects a large disc herniation, or if any neurologic compromise is present, MRI should be obtained immediately. Otherwise, for a more typical presentation of lumbar disc herniation that is not improving with nonsurgical treatment over a period of a few weeks, then an MRI should be obtained.

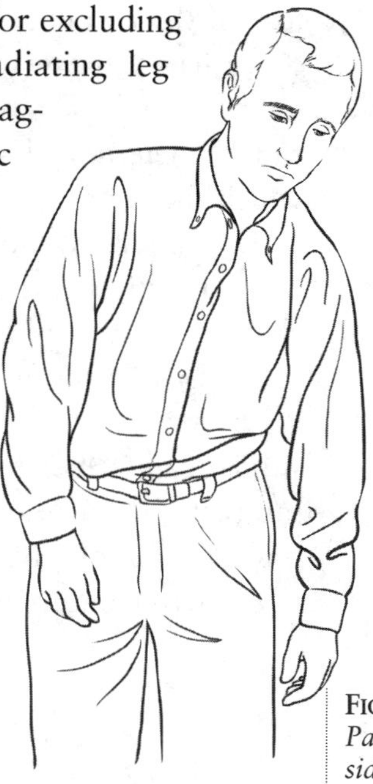

FIGURE 10.5
Patient tilting to the side because of nerve root compression

In chronic disc herniations, MRI will show loss of water content in a disc, but no evidence of an acute

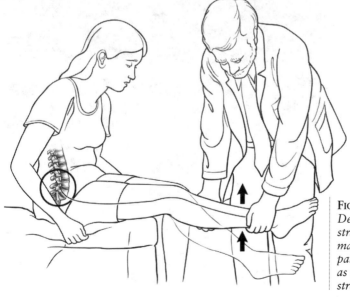

FIGURE 10.6
Demonstration of straight leg-raising maneuver. The patient's pain worsens as the affected nerve is stretched.

tear of the annulus. In acute disc herniation, on the other hand, the water content of the disc appears more normal. The relative water content of the disc can be determined with certain MRI sequences in which the water signal appears white (Figure 10.7).

Too often, radiologists interpret MRI studies without differentiating acute from long-standing changes in a lumbar disc. Thus, from the report alone, the physician does not know if the disc herniation developed recently or is longstanding. If MRI studies cannot be obtained, then a computed tomography (CT) scan is acceptable, although this provides less information about the disc itself.

Electromyography (EMG) and nerve conduction studies should be obtained if worrisome neurologic compromise is present. This helps to sort out the degree of nerve damage. For more straightforward cases of lumbar disc herniation that do not involve

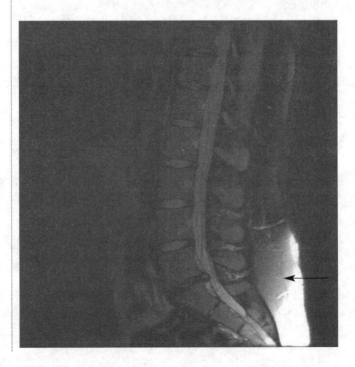

FIGURE 10.7
MRI film demonstrating an acute lumbar disc herniation at L5-S1.

numbness or weakness of the leg, EMG and nerve conduction studies are generally not necessary.

TREATMENT CONSIDERATIONS

Nonsurgical

Most patients with acute lumbar disc herniation can be treated nonsurgically. This is because the disc, over time, will gradually recede, thereby relieving pressure on other spinal elements. Even if a disc recedes completely, a disc that is herniated will never again be normal. Some water content will be lost, and subsequent degenerative changes may occur, leading to some loss of normal lumbar spine stability. Thus, long-term treatment must be directed at helping to restore spinal stability by other means.

Medications usually are indicated in the acute treatment of lumbar disc herniations. Anti-inflammatory drugs are quite useful in helping to alleviate inflammation and pain. Nonsteroidal anti-inflammatory drugs (NSAIDs) can be prescribed for 1 to 2 weeks. If pain is more severe, a corticosteroid may be prescribed for a 5- to 10-day course, instead of other anti-inflammatory drugs. Other medications include muscle relaxants if associated muscle spasm is present, or judicious use of narcotic analgesics for more severe pain.

Patients with acute lumbar disc herniation are generally too uncomfortable to undergo traditional physical therapy, although they may benefit from myofascial release or similar techniques. Acupuncture may be helpful, although the success of acupuncture for radiating leg pain is less than it is for low back pain per se. Spinal manipulation should not be utilized as an initial treatment for a lumbar disc herniation. Gentler mobilization techniques are appropriate. Epidural injections should be utilized if pain persists despite medication management and hands-on treatment. If pain is primarily in the leg as a result of a single nerve compression, then a selective nerve root injection is appropriate.

Once patients obtain reasonable pain relief, physical therapy should begin. Too often, patients arrive in a physical therapy facility, which is really no more than a mill, and they receive a "make, shake, and bake" approach in which multiple patients are treated simultaneously with a combination of modalities and cookbook-type exercises. More successful physical therapy employs a combination of manual techniques that help to restore muscle balance while allowing the therapist to understand relative areas of muscle weakness and imbalance. From there, a progressive spine stabilization protocol should begin. Over the long term, spine stabilization is the preferred treatment for patients who have suffered with lumbar disc herniation.

In conjunction with physical therapy, patients should be encouraged to resume or to return to exercise. If spine stabilization is successful, patients generally can return to any type of exercise.

Surgical

There are two absolute indications for immediate surgery in patients who present with a lumbar disc herniation:

- Bowel incontinence, bladder incontinence, or both that is attributable to the disc herniation.
- Progressive motor weakness or absolute motor weakness, attributable to the disc herniation.

If a disc herniation is quite large and primarily central, considerable compromise of the spinal canal can occur. This can then lead to a compression of the nerve roots that control the bladder and rectal region. If compression of these nerve roots is sufficient, patients become incontinent because the nerves are damaged (Figure 10.8). This is a neurologic emergency: Patients should be evaluated immediately by a spinal surgeon to undergo immediate spinal decompressive surgery.

Similarly, patients with rapidly progressive or absolute motor loss are at risk of permanent motor loss and should be evaluated immediately by a spine surgeon. Delay in surgical treatment for either scenario may result in permanent incontinence, muscle weakness, or both.

The third surgical indication is relative. For patients who have undergone good nonsurgical management, but who have refractory pain that is appropriate to the level of disc herniation, then surgery is indicated. The timing of surgery is a decision to be made between the patient and surgeon. Generally speaking, ongoing leg pain from an acute disc herniation should not persist beyond 3 months and, if nonsurgical therapy has failed

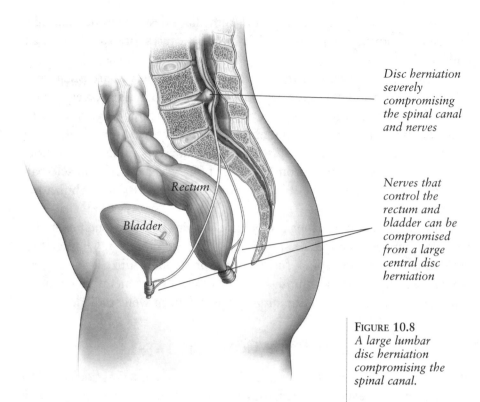

Disc herniation severely compromising the spinal canal and nerves

Nerves that control the rectum and bladder can be compromised from a large central disc herniation

FIGURE 10.8
A large lumbar disc herniation compromising the spinal canal.

to yield positive results by this time, then surgery is an appropriate option.

The medical risks of surgery must be considered carefully (see Chapter 7). As noted, the medical and rehabilitation risks of surgery are more substantial for patients undergoing spinal fusion when compared with patients undergoing laminectomy or diskectomy.

For a single-level disc herniation, surgery generally can be accomplished by way of a laminectomy or laminotomy with microdiscectomy. The herniated disc fragment is removed. Surgery is not curative for the remainder of the disc, and this disc will undergo some degenerative changes regardless of whether surgery has been performed. Successful surgery for a single-level disc herniation should lead to immediate cessation of pain. If pain relief is not immediate despite appropriate disc fragment removal, then possible physiologic causes of pain should be addressed.

Patients generally recover from surgery immediately and are discharged within 1 to 2 days. They often are walking the day of surgery, and resume full activity within weeks. As with patients who have undergone nonsurgical treatment, patients who undergo surgical treatment should ultimately work with a physical therapist who specializes in spine stabilization. These patients will benefit from a detailed analysis assessing muscle balance and strength, and should undergo a progressive spine stabilization protocol.

Unless other complications are present within the spine, such as multilevel degenerative changes or spondylolisthesis (discussed in Chapter 11), patients do not require spinal fusion. Some physicians utilize laser surgery, which essentially shrinks the disc and accelerates degenerative changes. The long-term success of laser surgery has not been well studied.

MIND–BODY CONSIDERATIONS

More often than not, patients and their treating clinicians focus on an inciting physical event that led to a disc herniation. Although this may provide part of an answer as to why the patient developed a disc herniation, the intent or perception surrounding the inciting event also may provide important clues. Psychological stress can lead to considerable physiologic changes in the body, including abnormal contraction of the lumbar spine musculature and even an abnormal spinal posture.

It is helpful for the patient to understand his perceptions around the time that pain developed. To do so requires either considerable trust between the patient and clinician, or the patient must be engaged in some type of mindful or meditative activity. Mindful and meditative activities allow individuals to move away from the distractions of day-to-day life and move into a place of turning inward, which may lead to a possibility of insight regarding various signals from the body.

Too often, we are unaware of day-to-day stressors. Then, when we become suddenly ill or injured, the focus turns to the injury or illness and not to our own sense of well-being versus our own sense of distress. This is not to say that all patients who develop a lumbar disc herniation have experienced stress. Rather, providing an opportunity for mindfulness may sometimes yield considerable beneficial results.

Illustrative Case

A 43-year-old woman presented with a 2-week history of severe right leg pain. She recounts that she had just returned from a trip and, as she was reaching overhead to remove some luggage, she felt a sudden pop in her lower back. Over the next 2 days, she developed increasingly severe pain in the right lower back. This pain was replaced by a severe, sharp, radiating pain in the posterior right leg, extending to the sole of the right foot. She could obtain relative relief lying on her back with her legs flexed. She was unable to sit or stand comfortably.

The initial physical examination revealed considerable restrictions with straight-leg raising and trunk flexion maneuvers. The neurologic examination revealed an absent reflex at the level of the right ankle, but was otherwise intact.

The patient was not very revealing in terms of other life circumstances. She was in considerable pain, and she was treated with a 6-day course of corticosteroids. She was also given a narcotic analgesic.

She did undergo a magnetic resonance imaging (MRI) of the lumbar spine, and this revealed a moderate disc herniation at the L5–S1 level, which compressed the right S1 nerve root. She was advised that nonsurgical management would be attempted, and she was to begin a course of physical therapy following treatment with corticosteroids.

The patient began to make some progress, but 3 weeks later called emergently. She developed the rather sudden onset of severe pain in the right leg, with numbness in the sole of the right foot and an inability to walk normally. Examination at that time was notable for showing an inability of the patient to toe raise in the right foot. Because of the neurologic changes, she had a repeat MRI study that revealed that the previous moderate disc herniation now was quite large and was compressing completely the S1 nerve root. Given the progression in the patient's symptoms, the size of her disc herniation, and the fact that she was failing nonsurgical treatment, spine surgery was recommended. She underwent a laminectomy at the L5–S1 level and developed immediate pain relief post operatively. Her strength returned over the next 2 months.

The patient began a course of physical therapy. She also became more revealing about circumstances surrounding her disc herniation. She had been visiting her dying mother in Florida, and she also was experiencing considerable difficulty with her teenage daughter. As a single mother, she felt that this stress in her life was enormous. She had little time for self-care and, when she was visiting her mother, she was essentially working nonstop, cleaning her mother's home, taking care of all paperwork, visiting her mother at any chance she could, and worrying about her daughter back home. It was upon her return home as she was lifting a piece of luggage that she developed her first symptoms.

Over the long term, the patient agreed to work with a psychologist for stress management and family counseling with her daughter. She also engaged in a physical therapy program. When she had a sense of spine stabilization, she began to participate in a regular program of yoga. She has remained faithful to this regimen since then and has remained asymptomatic.

Author's Note

This case illustrates the coexistence of mind and body imbalance in a patient who developed a lumbar disc herniation. Again, it is not always evident that patients have an imbalance both physically and emotionally, but it is worthwhile exploring this option. In addition, this case illustrates the important point that wholistic medicine embraces both surgical and mind-body considerations.

SUMMARY POINTS

- Lumbar disc herniation often develops gradually because of a genetic predisposition to degenerative disc changes.
- Sudden lumbar disc herniation can cause severe pain and sometimes causes leg numbness and weakness.
- Incontinence or severe leg weakness from lumbar disc herniation is a neurologic emergency demanding immediate decompressive spine surgery.
- Most cases of lumbar disc herniation can be managed nonsurgically; over the long term, most patients can return to full activity.
- Patients who develop lumbar disc herniation should try to reflect on significant life stressors that may predispose to spine imbalance.

CHAPTER 11

Lumbar Degenerative Disc Disease/Lumbar Spondylosis

CLINICAL PRESENTATION

Lumbar degenerative disc disease has no single, unifying presentation. A typical symptomatic patient has a clinical course of repeated bouts of low back pain, followed by long periods of pain relief. In this case scenario, a patient may describe a 10- or 20-year history in which he develops bouts of moderately severe low back pain, occurring once or twice yearly, sometimes severe enough to leave him bed bound, from which he gradually recovers to resume full activity. These bouts of pain may or may not be associated with radiating leg pain. The patient often is unaware of any particular inciting event to pain.

Although this may remain the pattern indefinitely, if the degenerative disc changes progress, then the patient can develop increasing symptoms. In some cases, a patient notes considerable morning stiffness or even severe pain on first standing in the morning. The morning pain may persist for a period of 30 to 60 minutes, until after he has fully showered and done some basic stretching exercises. Then, during the day, the patient feels relatively well. He may note that prolonged sitting, especially prolonged sitting in a car, is associated with an increase in symptoms, and getting in and out of the car may be particularly painful.

Morning stiffness and frequent bouts of pain also can be interspersed with more severe attacks of pain. This can manifest as a sudden, severe sense as if the back is locked; the patient becomes pitched forward or tilted to the side. If lumbar degenerative disc changes progress, then the patient may develop a pattern of more daily, situational pain, and may even develop a pattern of lumbar stenosis, which is described in Chapter 13.

The recurrence or increasing frequency of attacks generally leads a patient to seek medical help. This may be coupled with an increasing sense that the patient has become limited in certain activities, thereby diminishing quality of life.

Cause of Lumbar Degenerative Disc Disease

Degenerative disc disease primarily is caused by a genetically predetermined biochemical and metabolic alteration within the nucleus pulposus. The most notable changes occur between the ages of 30 and 50. Water content gradually diminishes as a result of the biochemical and metabolic shift, and the resultant drier and stiffer nucleus pulposus leads to fissures (tears). As a result, the entire disc complex begins to degenerate.

The sudden bouts of pain, which can develop intermittently, may be related to a sudden shift in the dynamic stability of the spinal joint. One

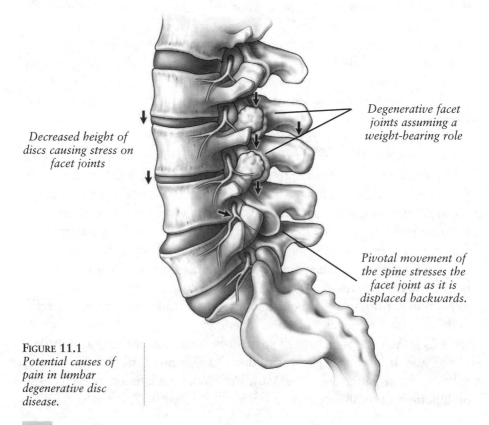

Decreased height of discs causing stress on facet joints

Degenerative facet joints assuming a weight-bearing role

Pivotal movement of the spine stresses the facet joint as it is displaced backwards.

Figure 11.1
Potential causes of pain in lumbar degenerative disc disease.

explanation may be that a larger tear develops within the annulus, associated with a disc herniation. This ultimately resolves without more specific treatment. Another possibility is that, as the disc loses its water content, the vertebral bodies approach each other, and the facet joints assume a more weight-bearing role (Figure 11.1). In this setting, the facet joints can suddenly become locked or irritated, causing sudden, severe, low back pain.

Another possibility is that, in the setting of degenerative disc changes, the spinal joint complex can become somewhat unstable and sudden, minor shifts can lead to irritation of pain-sensitive structures as well. When the lumbar disc is degenerative, the lumbar spine segments lose some stability. This means that bending forward or backward can be associated with abnormal movement of the lumbar vertebrae. The vertebrae may either rock back and forth or slide forward and backward (*pivotal movement*). In either case, pain-sensitive structures can become irritated. Lumbar degenerative disc disease also can be associated with spondylolisthesis, which is a fixed slippage of one vertebrae over another (Figure 11.2). This condition not only is associated with facet jamming, but may also lead to nerve compromise and spinal instability (see Chapter 12).

More progressive symptoms of degenerative disc changes are generally the result of minor instability of the lumbar spine coupled with facet irritation. The spine is no longer moving in a properly coordinated manner; in addition, the facet joints are becoming irritated because they are supporting the weight of the spine rather than acting as smooth, gliding joints. In addition, the lumbar musculature is generally poorly developed and cannot compensate for the lack of stabilizing forces of the lumbar disc. This cascade of events causes the patient to develop progressive symptoms.

PHYSICAL EXAMINATION

Patients with degenerative disc disease may reveal restriction of lumbar spinal flexion and extension. They also may develop pain at extremes of flexion and extension. Straight-leg raising maneuvers are generally unremarkable. A flattening of the normal lumbar curvature may be noted, secondary to prolonged maladaptive changes in the spinal segment and the spinal musculature. The neurologic exam is unremarkable.

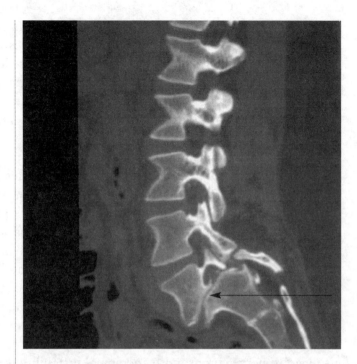

FIGURE 11.2
Reformatted CT film demonstrating forward spondylolisthesis at L5-S1.

IMAGING AND DIAGNOSTICS STUDIES

Plain radiographs of the lumbar spine reveal evidence of degenerative changes. The space between the disc may be narrowed and evidence of calcium deposits or osteophytes may be seen, which are the natural result of long-term, degenerative changes

Magnetic resonance imaging (MRI) will reveal evidence of loss of water content of the disc, and associated degenerative changes will be noted in the facet joints (Figure 11.3). Some narrowing of the spinal canal may be present, and there may be protruded disc material, which has become calcified over time. There may even be asymptomatic compression of nerve roots or evidence of spinal canal narrowing in the form of spinal stenosis (Figure 11.4). A computed tomography (CT) scan of the lumbar spine will reveal similar changes and may be more useful if greater detail is required for analysis of the facet joint. Electromyography (EMG)

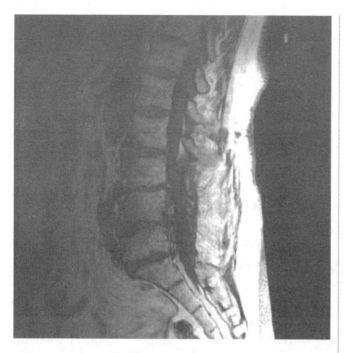

FIGURE 11.3
MRI film demonstrating lumbar degenerative disc changes.

and nerve conduction studies usually are not required, unless associated leg numbness or weakness is present. Occasionally, a bone scan is ordered as part of a general work-up for patients who have developed low back pain. A bone scan will reveal evidence of degenerative changes.

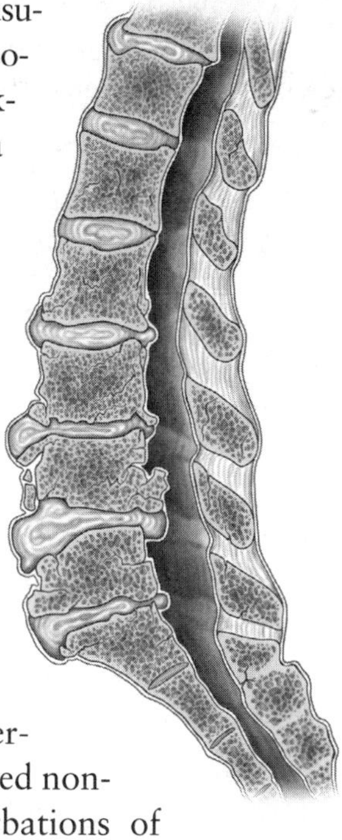

TREATMENT CONSIDERATIONS

Nonsurgical

In most cases, lumbar degenerative disc disease can be treated non-surgically. For acute exacerbations of

FIGURE 11.4
Lumbar degenerative disc changes with spinal canal narrowing.

147

pain, treatment with nonsteroidal anti-inflammatory drugs (NSAIDs) is appropriate. Such treatments generally last for 1 to 2 weeks. For a severe bout of pain, an oral course of corticosteroids may be indicated. Muscle relaxants may be helpful. Narcotic analgesics may be utilized to help with bouts of severe pain.

Spinal manipulation and acupuncture may be helpful for acute bouts of pain, but for the long term, the focus should be on manual physical therapy techniques and spine stabilization. In essence, patients generally develop a cascade of degenerative disc changes and muscular maladaptation; therapy must address the muscle imbalance and muscle weakness, then progress to spine stabilization. This is an attempt to allow the supporting musculature of the spine to help stabilize spinal movement.

In some cases, injections are indicated and can provide substantial relief. Patients may have prolonged back pain as a result of facet jamming or facet irritation and, a facet block may alleviate symptoms. Facet injections can be followed up by physical therapy. In some cases, degenerative disc disease is associated with partial herniation of disc material, with associated compression of the nerve route. A lumbar epidural corticosteroid injection or selective nerve root injection can help to alleviate symptoms. In all cases of therapeutic injections, treatment should be followed by a progressive course of physical therapy, as tolerated.

Surgical

Unless degenerative disc changes have progressed to the point of severe spinal stenosis (discussed in Chapter 13), or unless an associated neurologic compromise is present, most patients with lumbar degenerative disc disease can be managed nonsurgically. However, some patients develop multilevel degenerative changes and have associated spine instability. In this case, the spine will move repeatedly when the patient is in a forward flexed or backward extended position, causing a sudden jamming or irritation of pain-sensitive structures. If nonsurgical measures and physical therapy have not led to substantial pain relief, and if a good clinical correlation exists between the degenerative changes and the type of back pain that one might expect from such changes, surgery may lead to beneficial results.

If lumbar degenerative disc disease is associated primarily with some degree of spinal instability, then surgery must consist either of lumbar disc replacement or spinal fusion. In cases of back pain from degenerative, faulty lumbar discs, laminectomy alone may render the spine even more unstable. The medical risks of surgery must be considered carefully (see Chapter 7).

The success of spinal surgery depends on both the surgeon and the patient. Some patients have chronic low back pain without any clear precipitating or palliative features to the pain, but show some degenerative changes on imaging studies. When surgery is performed on such patients, failure is likely.

In contrast, other patients have clear clinical evidence of spine instability from a faulty lumbar disc. Such patients frequently develop considerable pain with sudden positional changes, such as getting out of the bed in the morning, getting into and out of a car, or suddenly misstepping. They also can develop sudden pain with certain twisting and bending activities. Walking on level ground generally leads to pain relief in such patients. If a good clinical history of such pain exists, with associated advanced degenerative disc changes on imaging studies, then disc replacement or spinal fusion may well lead to a good clinical outcome.

The surgeon determines whether to perform lumbar disc replacement, posterior fusion, or circumferential fusion. In part, this decision is based on the surgeon's experience with these procedures. The degree of spinal instability also influences the decision; patients with more severe instability will require spinal fusion.

Recovery from disc replacement surgery or spinal fusion surgery is more prolonged than it is from a simple laminectomy. The most prolonged recovery is from circumferential spinal fusion surgery. With any of these surgical techniques, patients may be required to wear a firm, plastic support brace for a period of 1 to 3 months following surgery. Physical therapy generally does not begin until at least 3 months following fusion, and it is extremely important to work with a skilled physical therapist. A modified program of spine stabilization should begin 3 to 6 months following surgery.

MIND–BODY CONSIDERATIONS

For many patients, lumbar degenerative disc disease is simply a fact of life. Whenever we consider mind–body interactions, we consider our genetic predispositions, and both internal and external environmental influences can modify such predispositions. In the case of lumbar degenerative disc disease, there may be little one can do with regard to the development of lumbar degenerative changes. In some cases, these changes may progress to lumbar stenosis, regardless of any intervention. However, it is still worthwhile to take a mind–body approach in lumbar degenerative disc disease.

Frequently, patients develop bouts of severe pain in situations similar to lumbar strain and acute lumbar disc herniation. That is, the bouts of pain develop in the setting of physical or psychological imbalance. In addition, patients may develop maladaptive strategies from the fact that they are predisposed to developing lumbar degenerative changes. Sometimes a mind–body approach simply means that we understand that our body is moving in a certain direction, and we need to adapt accordingly. Mind–body does not mean mind over matter. Mind–body refers to a sense of mindfulness and mindful listening to the body.

Over the long term, many patients with lumbar degenerative disc disease respond favorably to a program of both spine stabilization and meditative exercises such as yoga, Pilates, or t'ai chi.

Illustrative Case

A 55-year-old male presented to the office with complaints of increasing bouts of low back pain. He recalls that he developed his first episode of low back pain during his teenage years when he was playing high-school football. He missed two games, but otherwise was able to play up to 4 years. In college, he recalls having three or four bouts of sudden, severe low back pain that left him bed bound for several days at a time, but he then recovered uneventfully. In his 20s, he recalls being pain free for a period of many years but, for about the past 20 years, he has regularly developed attacks of low back pain, one to two times per year, each lasting a period of days to 1 to 2 weeks. For the past year, he has noticed morning stiffness, and he always has a sense of a vulnerable back. This has caused him to curtail some of his activities, such as weekend golfing and basketball.

The patient's family history is notable for a father, uncle, and two brothers who have had "bad backs." He is happily married, has three children who are healthy, and is a schoolteacher. Although he feels that his job is somewhat stressful, he does not feel that it is unduly stressful. He does not exercise on a regular basis; his days seem filled with activities, and he has made little time for self-reflection.

His musculoskeletal and neurologic examinations are largely unremarkable. Plain radiographs of the lumbar spine show evidence of disc space narrowing at L4–L5 and L5–S1. MRI of the lumbar spine reveals evidence of degenerative disc changes at L4–L5 and L5–S1, with associated facet changes and no significant spinal stenosis.

The patient was informed of his diagnosis, and he was not treated with any medication. He was referred to a physical therapist who specializes in spine rehabilitation. He was advised to try to find at least 30 minutes each day in which he engaged in some type of exercise, and he was to couple this with a back program. He faithfully followed through with the spine stabilization protocol, beginning a program of regular bicycle riding. Although he has low-grade symptoms, for the most part, he has been pain free and able to resume his weekend golf and basketball without compromise.

Author's Note

This case is quite typical for patients who suffer with lumbar degenerative disc disease. The intermittent attacks over time, with an increase in symptoms, are classic for the cascade of events that develop in this syndrome. Although this is called a degenerative condition, no compelling evidence shows that degeneration progresses to the point where patients will develop spinal stenosis or a progressively unstable spine. Most patients simply need to be mindful of their condition and make appropriate life adjustments.

SUMMARY POINTS

- Lumbar degenerative disc disease, also known as lumbar spondylosis, is primarily a genetically determined condition.
- Most patients with lumbar degenerative disc disease develop intermittent attacks of pain, followed by periods of complete pain remission.
- Most patients with lumbar degenerative disc disease can be managed nonsurgically. Such treatment should include a program of spine stabilization.

- Surgery is indicated for patients who develop spinal instability or progressive spinal stenosis.
- Lumbar degenerative disc disease does not necessarily cause low back pain; therefore, it is important to determine if low back pain is caused from degenerative discs or from another problem.

CHAPTER 12

Facet Pain

CLINICAL PRESENTATION

Facet pain is a result of the lumbar facet joint assuming an increasing weight-bearing role. Facet pain generally occurs in the setting of lumbar degenerative disc disease. Facet pain also can be associated with lumbar *spondylolisthesis*, which is a variation of lumbar degenerative disc disease, with associated slippage of one vertebra over another (Figure 12.1). Facet pain may be clinically indistinguishable from other types of mechanical back pain, but certain telltale symptoms and signs are present.

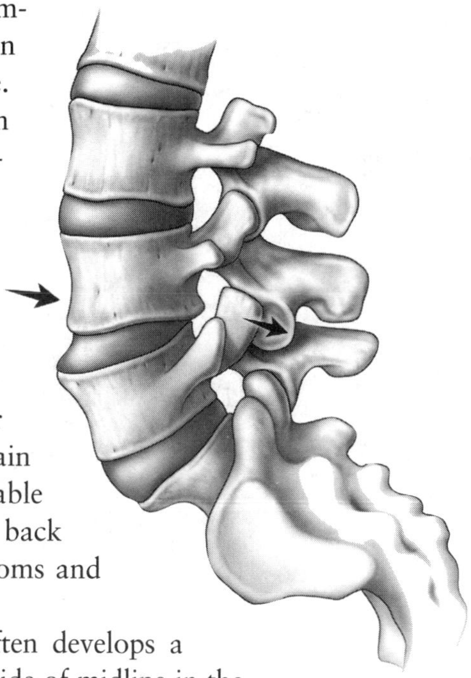

A patient with facet pain often develops a sudden, severe pain just to one side of midline in the lower back. Pain is relieved with trunk flexion, because this causes an unloading of the facet joints. Thus, as the patient bends forward, the facet joint opens up, which means it is no longer in a jammed position (Figure 12.2). Pain is worsened with trunk extension, especially with trunk extension and associated trunk rotation, because this causes more facet

FIGURE 12.1
Reverse spondylolisthesis of L4 on L5. The L4 vertebral body has slipped backward, and this has altered the normal position and function of the facet joint.

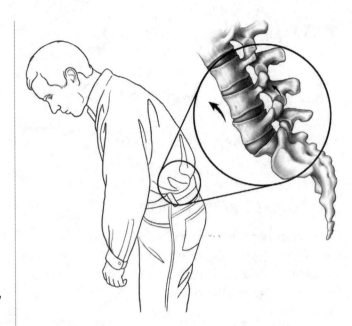

FIGURE 12.2
Opening (unloading) of the facet joint with forward bending.

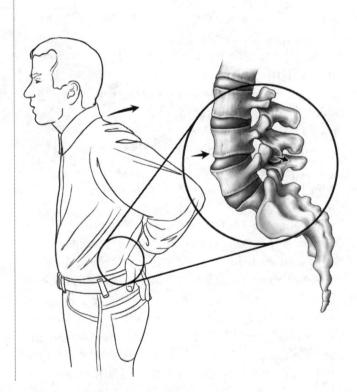

FIGURE 12.3
Facet jamming with trunk extension.

jamming (Figure 12.3). Pain may be referred into the buttock region and, rarely, into the leg.

Facet pain generally occurs intermittently, with attacks that can last for days at a time. In some cases, patients develop repeated facet jamming with sudden positional changes. This generally is associated with segmental lumbar instability.

CAUSE OF FACET PAIN

The facet joints are normally smooth, gliding joints that allow a directional movement of the spine based on facet orientation. In the lumbar spine, the facet joints allow trunk flexion and trunk extension. As the lumbar disc degenerates, the vertebral bodies approximate one another, leading to a loss of the normal space within the facet joints. Normally, the facet joint is lined with smooth cartilage, so that the space between the two facet segments allows for smooth, gliding movement of the spinal joint. The facet joint complex is part of the spinal joint, and thus entails two lumbar vertebral bodies. Thus, one can talk of the facet joints at the L4–L5 level, or the L5–S1 level, or any other two-level segment of the lumbar spine.

As the lumbar vertebral bodies approximate one another, the facet joints degenerate, and the pain-sensitive structures within the joint can become irritated (Figure 12.4). With sudden movement in a patient with lumbar instability, or with jamming of the facet joint in trunk extension, the patient can experience severe pain and sometimes will develop a reflex bending to the side or flexed forward posture.

PHYSICAL EXAMINATION

The patient with facet pain generally can bend forward without difficulty. Upon attempting to extend backward, especially with a rotation movement of the spine, well-localized pain develops. This pain arises from jamming and irritation of the facet joint with such movement. Sometimes, palpable tenderness is present just to the side of the lumbar spine, at the level of the irritated facet joint. Other aspects of the physical examination are largely unremarkable, unless severe, acute pain is present, in which case an associated muscle spasm is usually present. The neurologic examination is normal.

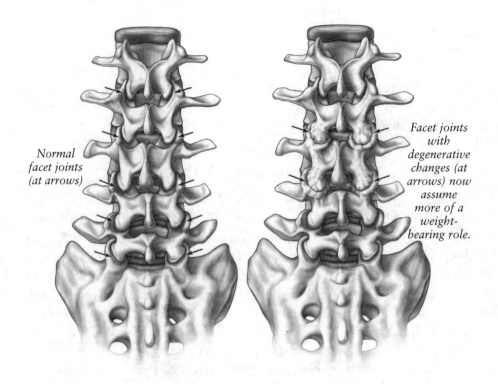

Normal
facet joints
(at arrows)

Facet joints
with
degenerative
changes (at
arrows) now
assume
more of a
weight-
bearing role.

FIGURE 12.4
*Back view of normal
and degenerative facet
joints. Note that the
degenerative facet
joints have essentially
no space for gliding
movement.*

IMAGING AND DIAGNOSTIC STUDIES

Plain radiographs of the lumbar spine will reveal evidence of degenerative facet changes, especially if an oblique view is obtained. Magnetic resonance imaging (MRI) and computed tomography (CT) scans will similarly reveal degenerative changes. Generally, the facet joints become hypertrophic. Associated spurring may be present; as the joint becomes more degenerated and stressed from assuming a weight-bearing role, the facet joint develops calcium deposits that can cause more dysfunction to the joint itself.

TREATMENT CONSIDERATIONS

Nonsurgical

Treatment for facet pain is very similar to treatment for degenerative disc disease. For acute bouts of pain, a nonsteroidal anti-inflammatory drug (NSAID) may be beneficial or, if pain is severe, a short course of corticosteroids may help to alleviate pain. Sometimes considerable reflex muscle spasm occurs with acute facet jamming. In this case, a muscle relaxant also will be helpful. Narcotic analgesics are appropriate for more severe pain.

Manual therapy techniques can be quite useful for facet jamming. Spine mobilization and careful spine manipulation may help to unload the facet joint. Manual physical therapy techniques similarly can help to unload the facet joints. Acupuncture may help to alleviate associated muscle spasm.

For the patient with prolonged pain that is anatomically referred to the facet joint, a facet injection may lead to considerable relief. In many ways, this injection is both diagnostic and therapeutic. A short-acting anesthetic, localized to the correct facet level, will lead to immediate pain relief. This can be coupled with a corticosteroid injection. If pain relief is obtained, then progressive physical therapy should begin, with a focus on facet unloading and spine stabilization.

Some patients may develop recurrent facet pain following a successful facet injection. If the diagnosis is secure, then a more definitive facet treatment by way of a rhizotomy may lead to more longstanding relief (Chapter 6). Rhizotomy procedures should be followed by progressive physical therapy to help the patient learn to stabilize the lumbar spine.

Surgical

Surgical treatment for facet jamming is similar to surgical treatment for lumbar degenerative disc disease (see Chapter 11). Most patients will not require surgery. For the patient who has refractory facet jamming, generally with associated spinal instability, then lumbar disc replacement or lumbar spinal fusion may be beneficial. Indications are similar to those for lumbar degenerative disc disease. The medical risks must be considered carefully (see Chapter 7).

MIND–BODY CONSIDERATIONS

Mind–body considerations for facet jamming are similar to those for lumbar degenerative disc disease, because most patients with facet degenerative changes are genetically predisposed to this anatomic development. Patients must be mindful that they have a degenerative lumbar spine, and they need to make appropriate adaptations, both in lifestyle and with regard to physical and psychological stress. Even patients with facet degenerative changes can have a full, active life, so long as they have made appropriate adaptations. Generally speaking, patients who follow through with a healthy exercise program and appropriate spine stabilizing exercises can do well over the long term. Stabilizing exercises such as yoga, Pilates, or t'ai chi also help patients to develop a good sense of centering and balance with regard to their lumbar spine in particular, and their well-being in general.

ILLUSTRATIVE CASE

A 65-year-old male came to the office with complaints of repeated bouts of low back pain. He has a longstanding history of intermittent low back pain but, for the most part, this pain has not limited him. For the past year, he has developed regular attacks of pain, which sometimes leave him debilitated. The pain typically occurs with back extension, and this has limited his ability to serve while playing tennis. When he develops attacks of pain, he obtains relief from sitting in a chair, especially if he flexes his trunk forward, or if he flexes his trunk from a standing position. Trunk extension leads to a marked exacerbation of pain.

The attacks of pain have become so frequent that the patient has become fearful of even performing minor exercise, and he has become quite cautious in his day-to-day activities. He has found that he has unconsciously developed an increasingly flexed forward posture, and he has developed an associated sense of tightness in his hamstring muscles.

The physical examination was notable for reproduction of low back pain with trunk extension, especially with trunk extension and right rotational bending. Trunk flexion was unremarkable, other than that the patient had rather taut hamstrings. He had a flattening of his normal lumbar curvature, and he was pitched forward slightly from a standing position. The neurologic examination was unremarkable.

The patient was diagnosed with lumbar facet jamming as a consequence of lumbar degenerative disc disease. A CT scan of the lumbar spine confirmed considerable lumbar facet hypertrophic and degenerative changes in conjunction with two-level lumbar degenerative disc disease, at L4–L5 and L5–S1. The patient was treated with a 2-week course of a nonsteroidal anti-inflammatory drug, coupled with physical therapy. Although he obtained some relief, he remained in pain. He then underwent a course of facet injections at the L4–L5 level, using a combination of Marcaine and corticosteroid medication. This led to substantial pain relief that allowed the patient to engage more fully in a progressive physical therapy program. He developed recurrent symptoms 6 months later and had a repeat set of facet injections. He has since remained relatively pain free, and he has been faithfully working out daily with a walking regimen and lumbar stabilization exercises.

Author's Note

This case is rather classic for progressive lumbar degenerative disc disease with facet jamming. Because the patient could not obtain relief with medication and manual therapy alone, a facet injection was appropriate. Because he did obtain good, prolonged relief with the facet injection, a rhizotomy procedure was not necessary. The patient's motivation and compliance with an exercise program has helped him in the long run, and he has remained rather asymptomatic. Sometimes simply taking the time, through exercise, to recognize the body's abilities allows an intuitive mind–body expression to unfold.

SUMMARY POINTS

- Facet pain usually develops in conjunction with lumbar degenerative disc disease. The pain results from the facet joint assuming a weight-bearing role rather than acting as a smooth, gliding joint.
- Forward bending often alleviates facet pain because this position opens up the facet joint.
- Treatment for facet pain is similar to treatment for lumbar degenerative disc disease. Patients may respond in particular to facet injections.

- Over the long term, spine stabilization exercises are important in helping to minimize future bouts of pain.
- Surgical indications for facet pain are similar to those for lumbar degenerative disc disease.

CHAPTER 13

Lumbar Stenosis

CLINICAL PRESENTATION

Lumbar stenosis means narrowing of the central spinal canal. Standing normally causes a narrowing of the lumbar spinal canal, and sitting somewhat enlarges the spinal canal. In patients with lumbar stenosis, the spinal canal is compromised, and upright activities such as standing and walking cause more canal compromise with associated symptoms.

Lumbar stenosis is a natural progression of lumbar degenerative disc disease. Some patients will give a history in which they have developed repeated attacks of pain over a period of many years, only to have the pattern of pain change. Other patients will have been relatively asymptomatic throughout most of their life until they begin to develop symptoms of lumbar stenosis.

The patient who is symptomatic from lumbar stenosis develops rather classic situational pain. Such a patient is comfortable sitting and is generally comfortable on first standing. However, with standing for a period of several minutes or with walking anywhere from half a block to many blocks, the patient develops increasing symptoms of low back pain. The back pain can become sufficiently severe that the patient must stop walking. Typically, the patient will either flex forward or sit down, obtaining almost immediate pain relief because these postures open up the spinal canal. Resumption of walking leads to recurrence of symptoms. Many patients relate how they can walk in a grocery store for a long period of time because they hold onto the grocery cart and can flex their trunk forward, thereby opening up the spinal canal.

Sometimes the patient will develop situational pain with standing and walking, but the pain will be referred down one or both legs. Flexing the trunk forward or sitting down will similarly alleviate symptoms almost immediately. The patient generally is comfortable lying down and generally does not awaken from pain in the middle of the night. If lumbar stenosis becomes more critical, the patient can develop associated leg numbness or weakness. If the spinal canal becomes quite compromised, then motor weakness and even bowel and bladder symptoms can develop, although this is unusual in lumbar stenosis.

As opposed to those patients who have arterial insufficiency in their legs, spinal stenosis patients can ride a bicycle or climb stairs without much difficulty. Arterial insufficiency, also known as *claudication*, means that the blood flow to the legs is diminished because of a blockage, usually from atherosclerosis, which is a fatty build-up within the artery. In arterial insufficiency, exercise involving the legs becomes impaired as the muscles, which demand more blood flow during exercise, become starved for oxygen since increased blood flow is unavailable.

Because riding a bicycle or climbing stairs involves flexing the trunk forward and opening the spinal canal, the patient with pure lumbar stenosis can tolerate these activities because his narrow spinal canal becomes more opened. The patient with arterial insufficiency develops symptoms based solely on whether the legs are demanding more blood flow because of an increase in muscle use from activity. Because both lumbar stenosis and arterial insufficiency tend to be medical conditions that develop in older patients, and therefore commonly coexist, it is important to make the distinction between these two conditions.

CAUSE OF LUMBAR STENOSIS

Lumbar stenosis is a natural extension of progressive lumbar degenerative disc disease. As the discs degenerate, bridging osteophytes may develop, and the facet joints may become hypertrophic. As noted in Chapter 11, degeneration of the discs brings the vertebrae closer together. The osteophytes are a type of calcium deposit that develops in response to the vertebrae approaching one another. As joints undergo hypertrophic changes, they become larger than normal; this increase in size is similarly a result of a calcium build-up that develops as a response to the facets approaching one another. The osteophytes and hypertrophic facet changes are a type of overgrowth phenomenon that narrows the spinal canal. As degeneration continues, the ligaments also can become hardened and thickened, producing further overgrowth changes. The end result is that a progressive encroachment occurs on the central spinal canal (Figure 13.1).

Normal spinal canal (from above)

The pain associated with lumbar stenosis may be from compromise of a lumbar nerve root, regional spinal blood flow, or both. Classic spinal stenosis pain develops in an upright posture, especially with walking, because blood flow in the spinal region increases. Because a competition for space in the spinal canal occurs, compromise of regional blood flow or nerve root develops; thus, assuming a more flexed-forward posture alleviates the symptoms.

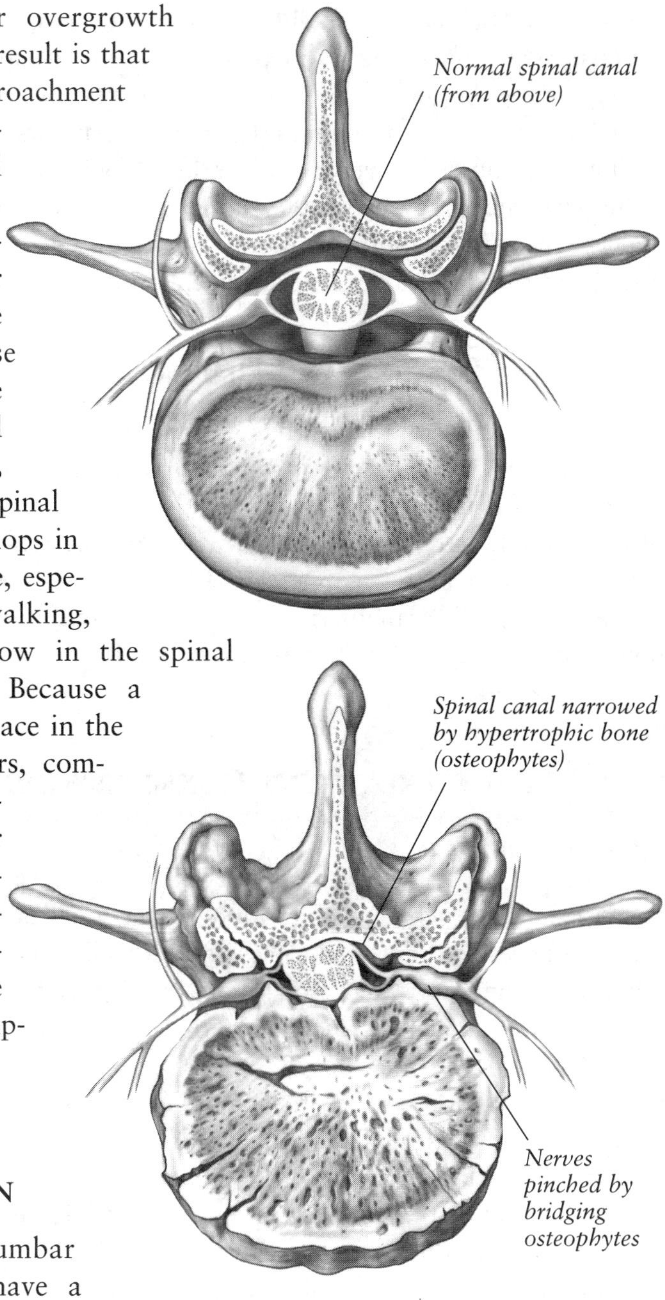

Spinal canal narrowed by hypertrophic bone (osteophytes)

Nerves pinched by bridging osteophytes

PHYSICAL EXAMINATION

Patients with lumbar stenosis usually have a flattening of the normal lumbar spine curvature. They are often pitched slightly forward when stand-

FIGURE **13.1**
Spinal canal changes in lumbar stenosis.

163

ing. Forward bending is usually without restriction, but backward extension usually is limited, either by pain or because the spine cannot move in such a manner because of the advanced degenerative changes. Usually, no palpable tenderness is present in the spine. In patients who have pain only, without numbness or weakness, the neurologic examination is normal. Otherwise, there may be subtle changes in reflexes, muscle strength testing, or sensory perception. Walking may be limited by pain, and patients often tend to pitch forward somewhat with more prolonged walking.

IMAGING AND DIAGNOSTIC STUDIES

Plain radiographs of the lumbar spine reveal evidence of degenerative changes, with disc space narrowing and osteophytes. Magnetic resonance imaging (MRI) is a more definitive study for lumbar stenosis. The health of the disc, the size of the spinal canal, and the relative location of the nerve roots can best be appreciated with an MRI study. A computed tomography (CT) scan of the lumbar spine may afford more accurate bony measurements, but provides less detail regarding the spinal canal and nerve roots.

TREATMENT CONSIDERATIONS

Nonsurgical

Because lumbar stenosis is situational pain, medication management is often unsuccessful. In essence, patients feel well when they are sitting and lying supine and only have pain while standing and walking. Because this is not an inflammatory condition, nonsteroidal anti-inflammatory drugs (NSAIDs) do not provide significant relief. However, subgroups of patients may improve. Narcotic analgesics are not indicated, because they generally do not help the situational pain while standing and walking and may leave patients feeling groggy otherwise.

Spinal manipulation is not indicated for lumbar stenosis, although gentle spine mobilization techniques may be helpful. Acupuncture may be helpful if maladaptive muscular responses contribute to symptomatology. Similarly, physical therapy and spine stabilization programs may be helpful if associated maladaptive responses cause symptoms.

Therapeutic injections by way of lumbar epidural corticosteroid injections may ameliorate symptoms, and sometimes this relief lasts for months. Occasionally, lumbar stenosis pain is associated with facet jamming, and a combination of epidural injections and facet injections may be indicated. If pain relief is sustained for months, patients can undergo repeat injections as needed; this treatment may be effective indefinitely. Sometimes, patients respond beneficially to therapeutic injections, become more active, and experience prolonged pain relief.

In some patients, epidural injections lead to considerable pain relief, but the pain recurs within weeks. Unfortunately, epidural injections should not be provided more often than 3 injections every 4 months and, in such cases, nonsurgical treatment options become limited. If patients have unilateral leg symptoms, selective nerve root injections may be more effective than lumbar epidural corticosteroid injections.

Surgical

Surgical indications for lumbar stenosis are somewhat similar to those for surgical indications for lumbar disc herniation (see Chapter 10). If the stenosis is critical and associated with bowel or bladder dysfunction or progressive motor loss, then emergency surgery is indicated, assuming the patient can tolerate such surgery medically. The difficulty with lumbar stenosis is that it is usually a disease of the elderly, similar to osteoarthritis of the hip and knees. Thus, this surgery may entail more serious medical risks (see Chapter 7).

A relative surgical indication for lumbar stenosis is that the patient has ongoing pain that has not responded to good conservative management. The classic patient who will generally do well with surgery is the patient who has responded quite beneficially to epidural corticosteroid injections, who has little medical risk, and who develops recurring pain weeks to months following the epidural injections. If spinal stenosis is limited to one or two spinal segments, then a decompressive laminectomy can be performed (Figures 13.2 and 13.3). In patients with more severe degenerative disc changes, or with evidence of spine instability, lumbar fusion is required in addition to decompressive laminectomy.

Some patients have severe, situational back or leg pain, but are not candidates for lumbar spine surgery. In select cases, a spinal cord stimulator may

Before decompressive laminectomy (from above)

Removed during laminectomy

Cross section of hypertrophic facet joints. Dotted lines show where bone will be removed during laminectomy.

Spinal canal narrowed and nerves pinched by bridging osteophytes. Dotted line shows where osteophytes will be removed during laminectomy.

After decompressive laminectomy (from above)

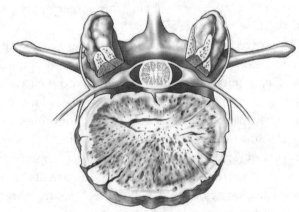

FIGURE 13.2
Lumbar stenosis changes before and after a laminectomy.

Hypertrophic bone from facet joints removed. Osteophytes removed. Spinal canal cleared and pressure taken off spinal canal and nerve roots.

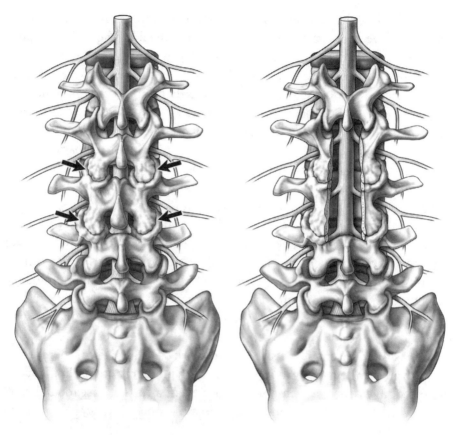

Hypertrophic facet joints before laminectomy (posterior view)

After decompressive laminectomy (posterior view)

be a viable alternative. The spinal cord stimulator may override the pain of the lumbar stenosis and, as long as the patient remains intact neurologically, such treatment may improve the quality of life considerably.

FIGURE 13.3
Posterior view (from behind) of lumbar stenosis changes before and after a laminectomy.

MIND–BODY CONSIDERATIONS

Lumbar stenosis is a result of a progressive lumbar degenerative disc disease. However, once patients develop lumbar stenosis, they do not necessarily develop progressive symptoms over time. Indeed, some patients develop worsening of spinal canal narrowing, but their symptoms improve. This latter consideration leads one to believe that other factors may be involved in the pain of spinal stenosis. In part, the body may develop adaptive changes.

Another possibility is that physiologic changes have occurred, and the pain threshold has changed. For example, there are occasions when the patient's perception of pain with lumbar stenosis can change according to the patient's underlying emotional sense of well-being. This is not universally the case, but the unexplained fluctuations of pain in patients who have lumbar stenosis suggest that physiologic pathways sometimes play a primary role in mediating pain. With this in mind, patients should be encouraged to engage in mindful activities, and issues that cause a sense of inner conflict should be addressed and resolved, if it all possible.

Many times, patients become increasingly discouraged when they develop progressive symptoms of lumbar stenosis, and they essentially lose their sense of hope. They become more chairbound, homebound, and socialize less and less, all out of fear of pain. This is a cycle that can lead to even more progressive maladaptive changes, both physically and psychologically. In addition to considering all other treatment options, patients should be encouraged either to work with a physical therapist or to perform some type of group exercise. Psychological counseling may be indicated. In essence, it is important to prevent a further cascade of symptoms, which can lead to a considerable loss of hope and associated depression in such patients.

ILLUSTRATIVE CASE

A 65-year-old retired male police officer presented with symptoms of progressive low back and leg pain. He recalls having suffered several injuries as a police officer and, on at least three occasions, he had severe low back pain lasting for a few weeks. He recovered from these injuries, and otherwise was doing well until about 3 years prior to presentation. At that time, he developed symptoms of some low back pain with walking. Over time, the patient developed increasing symptoms, to the point that he developed excruciating pain with walking more than two blocks. His pain was associated with a sense of tightness and sharp pain radiating into the back of the right leg. He had no leg numbness or weakness. He had no bowel or bladder symptoms. He had immediate relief of symptoms with sitting or lying down. He noticed that if he was grocery shopping and using a cart, he could walk for a more prolonged period of time, because he could pitch his trunk forward.

The physical examination was notable for showing a flattening of the normal low back curvature. A palpable slippage of the vertebrae in the low back was noted. The patient had limited ability to extend his trunk, and taut hamstrings limited his trunk flexion. His neurologic examination revealed a mildly diminished ankle reflex, but was otherwise intact.

Plain radiographs of the lumbar spine revealed a spondylolisthesis at L5–S1, meaning that slippage of the L5 vertebrae over the S1 bone occurred. Degenerative changes were noted at L4–L5 as well. Dynamic plain films of the lumbar spine—placing the patient in the forward flexion and backward extended position—revealed some movement of the L5–S1 spondylolisthesis with the spine fully flexed. MRI of the lumbar spine revealed degenerative changes at L4–L5 and L5–S1. Severe central stenosis was present at both levels. Electromyography (EMG) and nerve conduction studies revealed evidence of a bilateral S1 nerve root dysfunction, with no evidence of a peripheral neuropathy. Thus, the diminution in the ankle reflexes was attributable to pressure on the nerve roots from the spinal stenosis.

The patient was intolerant of all anti-inflammatory medications. He did not want to take narcotic analgesics or similar pain medications. He was extremely diligent in undergoing a program of physical therapy, which focused on manual muscle release techniques associated with progressive spine stabilization. Despite this, his situational symptoms persisted. He did undergo a series of lumbar epidural corticosteroids injections; each time he obtained excellent relief of symptoms, only to have the symptoms recur within 1 to 2 months.

After having exhausted all nonsurgical options, the patient agreed to meet with a spinal surgeon. Because of the instability at L5–S1, the patient required both spinal decompressive surgery and spinal fusion. Otherwise, he was at a risk of developing increasing lumbar instability following surgery. He successfully underwent lumbar spine surgery and fusion at L4-5 and L5-S1 and, other than mild low back pain, he is without further symptoms. He now walks 2 miles daily.

Author's Note

This case represents rather classic lumbar stenosis. This particular patient was quite diligent with his physical therapy work and was quite mindful of his body and psychological state while suffering from a progressive degenerative condition. He was an excellent surgical candidate, and he obtained excellent surgical results.

SUMMARY POINTS

- Lumbar stenosis is a degenerative condition of the spine that results in narrowing of the spinal canal.
- Lumbar stenosis causes pain when a patient is standing or walking, and pain is usually relieved when sitting down.
- Surgery is indicated for lumbar stenosis when bowel or bladder incontinence or severe leg weakness results from the stenosis. Surgery also may be performed when pain persists despite good nonsurgical management.
- Lumbar epidural corticosteroid injections sometimes provide relief for many months in patients with lumbar stenosis. If the relief is more short-lived, surgery may be necessary.
- It is important to consider secondary depression in elderly patients who feel a sense of hopelessness because of quality-of-life limitations secondary to symptoms of lumbar stenosis.

CHAPTER 14

Sacroiliac Pain

CLINICAL PRESENTATION

Sacroiliac pain refers to pain emanating from the sacroiliac region of the pelvis. Sometimes the pain is secondary to an inflammation of this joint (sacroiliitis), and sometimes the pain is from muscle imbalance around this joint. Sacroiliac pain is by no means straightforward. Very often, patients are diagnosed with sacroiliitis, despite no convincing clinical or radiographic evidence to support such a diagnosis.

As discussed in Chapter 2, the sacrum is a large triangular bone that lies just inferior to the lumbar spine. The sacrum also connects to the iliac bone, which forms part of the pelvis, by way of the sacroiliac joint (Figure 14.1). This is a relatively thin and immobile

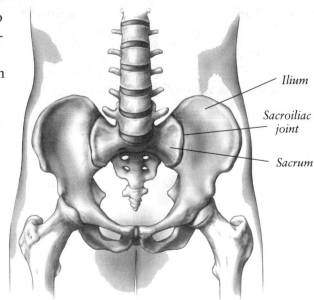

Ilium

Sacroiliac joint

Sacrum

FIGURE 14.1
Front view of the sacroiliac joint.

171

joint. During pregnancy, the sacroiliac joint actually enlarges somewhat, to help promote increased mobility during delivery.

Patients who have sacroiliac pain develop pain in the lower back, a few inches to the left or right of midline. Because this is a common area of referred pain from multiple causes of lumbar pain, many patients are given a diagnosis of sacroiliitis, but without underlying pathology in the sacroiliac joint per se.

Sacroiliitis is an inflammatory condition, usually in conjunction with an underlying rheumatologic disease. It can lead to severe pain in the low back region, especially on standing in the morning or on changing positions after having been in a prolonged sitting or supine position otherwise. As the pain progresses, it can limit all activities of daily living. Patients with sacroiliitis may develop radiating pain into the buttock and proximal back of the leg as well. No neurologic symptoms of numbness, tingling, or weakness are present.

As opposed to true sacroiliitis, patients with sacroiliac referred pain are usually suffering with a chronic strain of the deep rotator muscles of the lumbar spine. Because of this chronic imbalance, patients develop referred pain in the sacroiliac region. In addition, they have movement patterns that suggest instability in the sacroiliac region. Despite imaging studies that are either normal or show evidence of minimal degenerative changes, the patients carry a diagnosis of sacroiliitis, which is really a misnomer.

Some patients with a chronic pain syndrome or chronic myofascial pain also carry a diagnosis of sacroiliac pain. Both these conditions are discussed in Chapters 15 and 17. The ultimate course of sacroiliac pain depends on the underlying etiology.

CAUSE OF SACROILIAC PAIN

True sacroiliitis is a rheumatologic condition, and it may be a part of any of the following: ankylosing spondylitis, psoriatic arthritis, Reiter's syndrome, enteropathic arthritis, familial Mediterranean fever, rheumatoid arthritis, osteitis condensans ilii, or other rheumatologic conditions.

In some rheumatologic conditions, the sacroiliac joints become progressively narrowed and sclerosed, and generally an underlying inflammatory response is noted. *Sclerosis* of the sacroiliac joint means that the joint is becoming hardened and thickened, and the normal space within the joint is becoming progressively narrowed. This inflammatory and sclerosed response leads to activation of pain-sensitive fibers in the sacroiliac joint, thus becoming the anatomic basis of pain.

In noninflammatory, nonsclerotic sacroiliac pain, the pain is really from an imbalance of deep rotator muscles. The sacroiliac joint is simply an innocent bystander as this region of the lower back becomes dysfunctional. In this case, sacroiliac pain is a result of a lumbar strain, and lumbar strain can become chronic over time. In essence, an imbalance occurs in the deep rotator muscles of the lumbar spine and, because of this imbalance, a continual cycle of relative muscle weakness, muscle fatigue, and subsequent muscle strain occurs.

Pregnancy is a unique situation in which the pelvis must adapt to the enlarging uterus and to the eventual descent of the child through the birth canal. This adaptation is primarily accomplished through ligament relaxation secondary to hormonal changes. One of the most notable effects occurs in the sacroiliac joints; many believe that one prominent cause of low back pain during pregnancy is from the new mobility and relative instability of the sacroiliac joint. Following pregnancy, the hormonal levels that mediate ligament relaxation diminish, and the sacroiliac joint once again becomes more stable with associated limited movement.

PHYSICAL EXAMINATION

Patients with inflammatory sacroiliitis may have a stiffened appearance when walking and bending. Attempted movements of the hip, especially with external rotation, can be quite pain limited (Figure 14.2). The area of the back corresponding to the location of the sacroiliac joints may be quite sensitive to touch. In addition, various maneuvers in which the pelvis is challenged by thrusting it from either the front or behind can lead to referred pain in the sacroiliac region (Figure 14.3).

Patients with dysfunction of the sacroiliac region secondary to strain of the deep rotator muscles do not have such exquisite pressure tenderness and do not walk in such a stiffened manner. Trunk range of motion usually is uninhibited, but one can detect a subtle pivotal movement in the region of the sacroiliac joint when the patient moves from an extension to a full flexion position. Provocative maneuvers around the pelvis may cause some referred pain, but it is generally not excruciating pain. In addition, rotational maneuvers of the trunk against resistance can cause referred pain to the area of the deep rotator spinal muscles.

Imaging and Diagnostic Studies

Plain radiographs can be diagnostic in inflammatory sacroiliitis. To properly image the sacroiliac joint, a *Ferguson view* must be obtained. For the Ferguson view, the x-ray machine is tilted at an angle of about 15 to 30 degrees, allowing a better view of the sacroiliac joint. Sacroiliitis has characteristic stages, ranging from the most inferior portion of the joint becoming affected to a more diffuse sclerosis and bony proliferative change across the joint space, as the joint is remodeled with calcium deposits and inflammation. Ultimately, the entire joint space can be obliterated, and the ligament structure surrounding the sacroiliac joint may calcify.

A computed tomography (CT) scan of the pelvis can delineate these sclerosing changes further. Plain films and CT scans provide more useful details than do magnetic resonance imaging (MRI) studies with regard to sacroiliitis. If

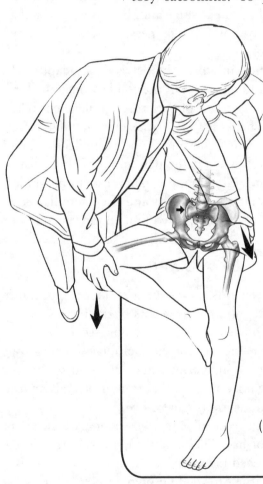

Figure 14.2
Sacroiliac pain from external hip rotation.

sacroiliitis is detected, then rheumatologic testing must be performed. This is best done under the guidance of a rheumatologist.

TREATMENT CONSIDERATIONS

Nonsurgical

If sacroiliac dysfunction is a result of inflammatory sacroiliitis, the underlying cause of the inflammation must be addressed. This is often a result of an autoimmune disease and, in this case, a combination of nonsteroidal anti-inflammatory drugs (NSAIDs)

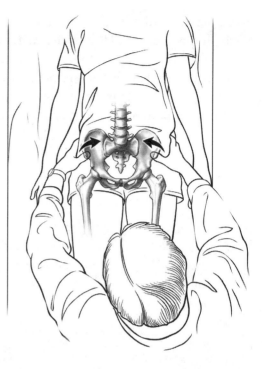

FIGURE 14.3
Sacroiliac pain from a pelvic thrust maneuver.

plus other disease-modifying agents may be required. Therapeutic injections, including an anesthetic plus corticosteroid directed into the sacroiliac joint, can provide short-term, considerable pain relief. These injections may be used in conjunction with other disease-modifying agents. Once the pain is under reasonable control, then manual physical therapy is also a good adjunct, and such therapy can help balance the pelvic musculature with pelvic strengthening.

In noninflammatory sacroiliac dysfunction, the underlying muscle imbalance must be addressed. Short-term use of an NSAID may help to alleviate symptoms. For severe pain referred to the sacroiliac region, a therapeutic injection into the sacroiliac joint may be considered. Acupuncture, spinal manipulation and mobilization, and manual physical therapy are all beneficial in this scenario. Ultimately, an aggressive course of spinal stabilization is required to help minimize future episodes of sacroiliac dysfunction.

For pregnant patients, a simple *trochanteric belt* sometimes leads to considerable relief. This is an elastic, supportive belt that is placed under the protuberant abdomen to help stabilize the pelvis and sacroiliac region. Pelvic floor and simple spine stabilization exercises should be used in conjunction with a trochanteric belt.

Surgical

In rare cases, the sacroiliac joint can be fused surgically. This should only be done in cases of a progressive, inflammatory disease with partial destruction of the sacroiliac joint. The sacroiliac fusion should not be considered in cases of noninflammatory sacroiliac dysfunction.

MIND–BODY CONSIDERATIONS

For patients who have an underlying rheumatologic disease, it is extremely important to try to engage in some form of mind–body awareness. This is not specific for a rheumatologic condition, but rather affords considerable benefit for patients with any chronic disease state.

Clear and convincing evidence shows that a relationship exists between the state of the nervous system and the responsiveness of the immune system. This is not to say that a direct causal link exists. However, a program of exercise and mindfulness, coupled with stress reduction, can help to optimize the body's neuro-immunologic response. It is certain that there exists an intimate coupling between the emotional brain and the immune system, and we are just beginning to understand the applications of this coupling. To date, compelling data demonstrate the usefulness of mindfulness with regard to helping patients who suffer with autoimmune diseases.

In patients with noninflammatory sacroiliac dysfunction, we again face a problem of physical imbalance and, where there exists physical imbalance, there is often an associated emotional imbalance. Chronic stress and chronic misuse or overuse of the body have emotional counterparts, and all take a toll on the ability of the body to compensate over the long term. Programs of stress reduction and insight-oriented behavior may be quite helpful in such patients, and long-term, meditative exercises that promote body awareness complement spine stabilization exercises.

ILLUSTRATIVE CASE

A 30-year-old woman presented with a history of refractory low-back pain. Her past medical history was notable for a diagnosis of ulcerative colitis, which is an autoimmune, inflammatory disease affecting the colon, with frequent bouts of abdominal pain, abnormal bowel movements, and bloody stools. The diagnosis of ulcerative colitis was delayed for over 1 year, because the patient's parents simply thought that she was anxiety-prone, and they did not take her symptoms seriously. Although the patient herself has always admitted to some relationship between her underlying stress and her ulcerative colitis symptoms, she also felt that the attacks of pain and bloody diarrhea were beyond any simplistic relationship to her underlying stress.

Following the diagnosis of ulcerative colitis, the patient began a program of diet change and treatment with azulfidine. Azulfidine is a disease-modifying medication that helps to diminish the abnormal autoimmune, inflammatory response. Early in the course of treatment, she had a severe flare of bloody diarrhea and was given a course of oral corticosteroids. Ultimately, her ulcerative colitis symptomatology became well-controlled.

For about 1 year prior to her current presentation, she had increasingly severe symptoms of pain in the sacroiliac region, radiating into the buttock, but not into the legs. She was quite stiff in the morning, and felt increasingly limited with regard to her ability to exercise and engage meaningfully in day-to-day activities. She had undergone chiropractor treatment for 6 months, to no avail. She had plain radiographs of the lumbar spine performed by the chiropractor, who told her she had a "subluxation" of her vertebrae and that repeated spinal manipulation would ultimately correct this subluxation.

On initial examination, radiographs were reviewed. They were unremarkable other than for some mild straightening of the normal lumbar curvature. No subluxation was evident. She had several signs referable to the sacroiliac joint, and all provocative pelvic thrusting maneuvers led to a marked reproduction of her pain. Her neurologic exam was unremarkable. Radiographs of the pelvis using Ferguson views revealed sclerosis of both sacroiliac joints, with some associated bone loss. The patient was diagnosed with sacroiliitis, and her case was discussed with the treating gastroenterologist. She underwent rheumatologic evaluation, which was otherwise unremarkable.

Because the patient had severe pain, she underwent bilateral sacroiliac injections and obtained good relief. She underwent a more prolonged course of manual physical therapy with a focus on spinal stabilization and more aggressive treatment of her underlying inflammatory bowel disease. In addition, the patient began a regular program of yoga. Although she still has flares both with regard to the intestinal dysfunction and her lower back, she overall feels improved.

Author's Note

Inflammatory bowel disease is often underdiagnosed and, depending on the mindset of the family and physician, may be misdiagnosed as functional or irritable bowel syndrome. On the other hand, some patients with functional or irritable bowel syndrome are overdiagnosed with inflammatory bowel disease. Either diagnosis requires skillful analysis by a gastroenterologist. Some patients with chronic diseases develop a lifestyle of frequently being ill and frequently complaining, and sometimes their complaints are not taken seriously. Such was the case for this patient, both with regard to her intestinal dysfunction and later with regard to her lower back dysfunction.

It is not clear whether the underlying sacroiliitis in conjunction with inflammatory bowel disease is related to the same autoimmune process causing inflammatory bowel disease, or is a result of abnormally absorbed antigens from an inflamed intestine. (*Antigens* are proteins that the body may "attack" as an invader, thus causing more inflammation.) In either case, treatment of the underlying bowel disease is required, and if the patient remains symptomatic, then the treatment paradigm must change. Even as this is done, sacroiliac dysfunction itself can be addressed directly, which can help ameliorate symptoms.

SUMMARY POINTS

- Sacroiliac pain results from dysfunction of the sacroiliac joint region, but is not necessarily caused from sacroiliitis, which is an inflammation of the sacroiliac joint.
- Low back pain is frequently misdiagnosed as sacroiliitis.
- Except during pregnancy, the sacroiliac joint is essentially immobile.
- Treatment of sacroiliac pain varies considerably, depending on whether or not true sacroiliitis exists.
- Sacroiliitis is often a result of an underlying rheumatologic condition, which must be addressed in and of itself.

CHAPTER 15

Myofascial Pain

CLINICAL PRESENTATION

Myofascial pain, sometimes known as *myofascial pain syndrome* or *regional myofascial pain*, is a condition whose diagnosis is based on clinical findings. Myofascial pain is defined as a pain syndrome that exists in a region of the body, and that is not caused by a physical problem within the spine or nerves. The muscles and supporting muscle tissues may be tender or in spasm, but these changes are not the primary cause of the pain. The pain of myofascial pain is thought to originate from abnormal signals within the nervous system. As such, myofascial pain is a type of neuropathic pain.

No imaging or diagnostic tests prove the diagnosis. Some believe that myofascial pain is simply a psychosomatic pain syndrome, but this is not in keeping with the scientific and medical literature available. In other words, myofascial pain is a well-established clinical entity that is too often underdiagnosed or misunderstood by physicians and other health care practitioners. In this setting, the clinician may simply prefer to state that no medical basis exists for pain rather than admit that he does not understand the basis for the pain.

Myofascial pain generally presents in one region of the body and, with regard to the lower back, myofascial pain can present as a diffuse low back pain, as a regional pain on one side of the back or the other, or as pain with radiation into the gluteal and proximal leg musculature.

Patients who suffer with myofascial pain may experience exacerbations and remissions of pain. Very often, no clear precipitating or palliative features to these exacerbations and remissions are present. Patients often remark that the pain "seems to have a life of its own." This distinguishes myofascial pain from more mechanical and situational pain syndromes such as a lumbar disc herniation or lumbar stenosis.

Pain often is described as deep, aching, and sometimes burning. Pain frequently awakens the patient from sleep. The patient often feels somewhat better when he is more physically active.

Myofascial pain may be the result of repetitive trauma or overuse, or it may be a response to a more singular traumatic event. For example, some patients may develop myofascial pain following a sudden accident. The difficulty in making this diagnosis is that the severity of the trauma per se does not predict whether someone will develop myofascial pain. For example, a minor car accident may become the inciting event for severe myofascial low back pain. Thus, it is the patient's response to the trauma or repetitive traumas that determines the outcome, and not the physicality of the trauma in and of itself. This response is both physical and physiological, which means that the response has to do with the musculoskeletal system and the emotional–cognitive processing system, that is, the mind–body.

Myofascial pain may exist as a continuum with another condition known as *fibromyalgia*. Fibromyalgia is a more diffuse pain syndrome, affecting multiple joints or multiple muscular trigger point areas in the arms, legs, neck, and trunk. Some patients seem to move in and out of a fibromyalgia presentation and myofascial pain presentation over time.

Myofascial pain can coexist with other musculoskeletal conditions. For example, some patients may have radiographic evidence of lumbar stenosis, but their clinical presentation suggests a myofascial pain syndrome. Similarly, patients may have a herniated lumbar disc, but they do not present with the characteristic symptoms of mechanical pain from a disc herniation. Sometimes, the body responds to the lumbar stenosis or herniated disc in such a manner that it develops a transformed pain syndrome. Clinicians must learn to rely on making a firm diagnosis based on the clinical presentation. Imaging studies alone are insufficient to make a diagnosis and treatment plan.

Myofascial pain can be a short-lived response to a traumatic event, or it can become a more chronic condition. When myofascial pain becomes chronic, other markers of disability often are present, from a psychological, social, and physical point of view, and all these factors must be considered in treating the patient.

CAUSE OF MYOFASCIAL PAIN

Various explanations are given for myofascial pain, but no one unifying explanation exists for this condition. With regard to the lower back, the muscles involved often include the deep rotator muscles, the iliopsoas, the gluteal muscles, and piriformis. Tenderness to palpation may be present, but this is not always the case. The muscles generally have a maladaptive state, with decreased flexibility, abnormal consistency, pain with contraction, and a hypersensitive response to internal and external triggers.

Myofascial pain is a neuropathic pain condition, meaning its genesis lies in a dysfunction of the nervous system. Myofascial pain has a remarkable biochemical and physiologic similarity to migraine. Migraine is a disorder of the trigeminal vascular complex—the nerves and blood vessels that innervate the brain and head. In migraine patients, a hypersensitivity exists in this entire system, with abnormal "pacemaker" activity in the brainstem. This results in pain signals and regional inflammatory chemicals being generated, despite the fact that no localized trauma is present to cause such pain. In some migraine patients, the pain becomes transformed into a chronic, daily headache.

Myofascial pain has a similar presentation. Abnormal pacemaker activity occurs in the brainstem, and a hypersensitivity response is triggered between the brainstem and the region of the spinal cord that mediates the local pain response. Abnormal pacemaker activity means that a particular brain circuit sends signals unusually fast or slow. The brainstem pacemaker is commingled with parts of the brain that sustain emotional and cognitive activity. As a result, patients who suffer with myofascial pain may note a relationship between uncompensated stress and pain response.

The serotonin and norepinephrine pathways are particularly involved in the expression of myofascial pain. The serotonin and norepinephrine centers are located in the brainstem and project widely to multiple brain and body areas. Serotonin and norepinephrine are the chemical mediators of multiple physical expressions, including depression, anxiety, and irritable bowel syndrome. Thus, it also comes as no surprise that patients who suffer with myofascial pain may also suffer with depression, anxiety, irritable bowel syndrome, migraine, or some combination thereof.

PHYSICAL EXAMINATION

The musculoskeletal examination may be rather unremarkable in a patient who presents with myofascial pain. At times, areas of specific trigger points may be present, and pain with resistance to certain trunk movements may be present. The neurologic examination is normal. Indeed, it is the paucity of physical findings that has led some clinicians to doubt the existence of myofascial pain and to suggest to a patient that the pain must be "in your head."

IMAGING AND DIAGNOSTIC STUDIES

Patients with myofascial pain have no abnormalities in imaging or other diagnostic studies that correlate with or explain their pain. Incidental abnormalities may be present, and this is often the case when patients undergo an evaluation. For example, a patient who presents with 1 year of low back pain and who undergoes a lumbar spine magnetic resonance imaging (MRI) may be told that he has degenerative discs or even a disc herniation. Because of these abnormalities, and because there is no other "objective" explanation otherwise for pain, the patient and clinician may then embrace the idea that the pain is anatomically generated from these abnormal discs. This can then lead to a cascade of unsuccessful treatments directed at these discs.

TREATMENT CONSIDERATIONS

Nonsurgical

Patients with myofascial pain benefit from a multidisciplinary approach. The first and sometimes most important aspect of treatment is to evaluate the patient and to assure him that he does have real physical pain. Too often, patients with myofascial pain have sought numerous medical opinions, have been told that nothing is wrong, and then begin to doubt themselves, the medical profession, or both.

Routine physical therapy often exacerbates myofascial pain. Physical therapy is too often a simplistic combination of ultrasound, electrical stimulation, and cookbook-type exercises. If the abnormal tension, contractility, and hyperresponsiveness of the musculature are not addressed, then exercises can worsen the pain.

Skilled hands-on therapy, including spinal manipulation, physical therapy with a focus on myofascial release and craniosacral technique, and acupuncture can help to reshape the maladaptive muscular response of myofascial pain. This type of treatment in and of itself can be extremely beneficial.

Patients often benefit from medication. One of the most successful medications for myofascial pain is amitriptyline, which is an old-fashioned antidepressant medication that nonspecifically increases the availability of norepinephrine and serotonin (see Chapter 5). This medication promotes sleep, and patients with myofascial pain are often sleep deprived. Amitriptyline generally is prescribed in a low dose, 10 mg to 25 mg, which is lower than the therapeutic dose required to treat depression.

Anticonvulsants sometimes are useful in treating myofascial pain, especially when the pain has a burning component and when the pain has become severe. The choice of anticonvulsant depends on other symptoms that the patient is experiencing. Some anticonvulsants help to promote sleep, some anticonvulsants are associated with weight loss, and others are associated with weight gain. Newer-generation antidepressant medications also serve as a useful adjunct in treating myofascial pain, because very often an associated anxiety, depression, or both are present. In addition, numerous well-designed scientific studies have demonstrated the efficacy of newer-generation antidepressant medication in alleviating neuropathic pain.

Narcotic analgesics generally are avoided unless the pain is refractory. Tramadol may be a useful alternative to traditional narcotic analgesics. Nonsteroidal anti-inflammatory drugs (NSAIDs) have little role in the treatment of chronic myofascial pain. Muscle relaxants may be quite effective in some patients, especially when abnormal hypercontractility of the involved musculature occurs.

Psychological counseling, group therapy, or both may be an important intervention in patients suffering with myofascial pain, especially those who have been suffering chronically. In such cases, a complex interplay often exists between emotions and pain, or there may simply be a secondary depression that must be addressed. As stated earlier, patients with chronic pain who are also suffering with depression will not improve unless depression is adequately managed.

Therapeutic injections have little role in myofascial pain, other than the judicious use of trigger-point injections. An over-reliance on trigger point injections should be avoided, and such injections should be coupled with manual therapy. Botulinum toxin (Botox) injections have been tried with myofascial pain, but their efficacy is unclear.

Exercise is exceedingly important for patients who suffer with myofascial pain. However, the exercise should be a part of a comprehensive, multidisciplinary approach, and should be tailored to the patient's overall clinical presentation. Meditative exercises such as yoga, t'ai chi, and Pilates benefit many patients suffering from myofascial pain. Other forms of exercise, such as walking, swimming, or biking, may be well tolerated and ultimately beneficial, once the pain cycle is under better control.

Surgical

There is little role for surgical treatment in myofascial pain. Too often, patients with myofascial pain undergo surgery for degenerative lumbar discs or similar conditions, only to have increased pain following surgery because surgery does not address the cause of pain. In essence, surgery is yet another trauma that the body must adapt to, and patients with myofascial pain already have a maladaptive response to trauma. Thus, pain can worsen substantially following such surgical intervention.

Spinal cord stimulator placement also should be avoided in myofascial pain, unless patients have an extraordinarily well-localized pain and have exhausted all other aspects of pain management. Even in this case, patient selection must be exceedingly careful. Certain patients, having exhausted all other aspects of pain management, may become dependent on narcotics coupled with a systemic intolerance to these medications. In such cases, placement of a morphine pump may be indicated.

MIND–BODY CONSIDERATIONS

A mind–body approach is extremely effective in managing patients with myofascial pain. This is a classic pain syndrome in which a well-defined relationship exists between the emotional response and the pain response.

Many patients who suffer with myofascial pain have undergone physical trauma, but the psychic response to trauma often is underexplored. It is not the traumatic event per se that determines the onset of myofascial pain, but the patient's interpretation and insight into the traumatic event.

Because myofascial pain can be worsened by emotions and perceptions, meditative techniques, relaxation techniques, and biofeedback help patients to gain insight into the relationship between pain and emotions. At a deeper level of insight, patients with myofascial pain may come to understand a connection between a repressed or disassociated conflict that has no apparent peaceful reconciliation and that has led to a chronic, low-grade, post-traumatic stress-type behavior. Such patients often are exceedingly compulsive and well organized, to the point that every aspect of their day is placed in order. By doing so, patients have developed a sense of order that compensates for the disorder within.

With this latter point in mind, it is interesting to come to an understanding of the patient's perception of where he was at the time the myofascial pain began. Something such as a minor car accident, in which the physicality of the event becomes the focus of treatment and medical–legal work, may have profound psychic implications. Sometimes the car accident happens when the patient is physically and emotionally at a point of exhaustion. This trauma represents the "final blow," and the patient begins to decompensate. If pain develops, this may become the focus of the decompensation, because this expression may be psychologically preferable to becoming a witness to the emotional pain. This is not to state that all patients who suffer with myofascial pain have such a simplistic mind–body explanation. However, to resist exploring such a possible connection may limit avenues of appropriate treatment.

ILLUSTRATIVE CASE

A 35-year-old woman presented to the office with complaints of chronic low back pain. She dated her history to 3 years earlier, when she was stopped at a red light and her car was struck from behind by a truck. Her 3-year-old daughter was in the back seat of the car, and the patient feared that her daughter's life was in danger. She does not recall having any immediate symptoms of pain. She got out of the car, took care of her daughter, and immediately brought her to the hospital. The daughter recovered from minor injuries.

Within days, the patient developed increasing symptoms of low back pain. The pain radiated diffusely across her low back and somewhat into the right buttock region. She sought chiropractic treatment and, although this provided short-term relief, she was no better, even after having undergone treatment three times weekly for 6 months. She sought orthopedic surgery treatment and was prescribed NSAIDs for 1 month, coupled with routine physical therapy. She did not improve. She then underwent treatment with a naturopath, who treated her with various herbs and other nutraceuticals. After a course of prolonged treatment, the patient noted no improvement.

On a day-to-day basis, the patient had chronic pain. She awakened with pain, and pain could awaken her from her sleep. She described the pain as a deep ache, with an occasional deep feeling of warmth. She felt somewhat better, or was less distracted by the pain, when she was active during the day. Toward the end of the day, the pain became excruciating, to the point that she was often in tears. She was a full-time homemaker and, after she had finished her daily chores, which included cooking dinner, cleaning, and putting the child to bed, she herself fell asleep, exhausted. She had no meaningful sexual relations in over 1 year.

Plain radiographs revealed a straightening of the normal curvature of the lumbar spine. A magnetic resonance image (MRI) of the lumbar spine revealed disc bulges at L3–L4 and L4–L5. The MRI study had been officially read as revealing disc herniations at these two levels and, of note, the facility that produced the report was often utilized by physicians who work with lawyers involved in medical–legal work.

Physical examination revealed trigger point areas of tenderness in the sacroiliac and right gluteal region. The patient had full mobility and a normal neurologic exam. She was diagnosed with myofascial pain, and a multidisciplinary treatment program was recommended. She initially began treatment with amitriptyline 10 mg and physical therapy, which focused on myofascial release and craniosacral technique. Group therapy was recommended. The patient was to be re-evaluated after several weeks of this approach.

Following 3 weeks of physical therapy treatment, the patient called emergently. During one of the physical therapy sessions, she developed an extraordinary cathartic response. While she was lying still, something she had not done in over 2 years, she became overwhelmed with a flood of previously repressed emotions and began to sob, almost uncontrollably. This catharsis helped the patient to gain insight into her state of being.

She was at a loss with regard to her own career outside the home, which she had placed on indefinite hold when she became a mother. She felt no sense of emotional bonding or support from her husband, and she felt increasingly isolated from her family and friends. The accident itself was quite forceful, to the point that her car was totaled. She is not even certain how she survived the accident without any broken bones, and she still develops considerable inner anxiety when she thinks about the possibility that her daughter could have died as a result of the trauma.

As she began to reconcile with these emotions, she came to understand that she had gone into a state of hyperalertness coupled with considerable anxiety, but that she completely disassociated from these feelings. She came to understand that the physical pain might have been a preferred expression to her underlying, deep-seated emotional pain. This insight allowed the patient to verbalize her feelings in group therapy and, during therapy, she came to understand that she was not alone with her feelings. She saw the clinical utility of group therapy, and she was guided into becoming a witness to her feelings.

The patient ultimately began a course of more intense individual psychotherapy. She and her husband began marriage counseling. She began a mindful exercise program in the form of yoga. Over a period of many months, her pain resolved, she was weaned from medication, and she developed a much greater sense of well-being.

Author's Note

Myofascial pain is a classic mind–body condition. Patients with myofascial pain suffer with real, physical pain. We must always remember this point. The physical suffering is based on dysfunction of the nervous system and is not imaginary. Understanding the nervous system dysfunction, or modulating its expression, holds the key to managing successfully the patient with myofascial pain.

In this example, the patient's insight into the connection between her emotional pain and its physical expression allowed her to begin a healing journey. She developed this insight in the setting of a trusting environment, and she sensed deeply that she could explore her emotions without being judged. Nonjudgment allows the exploration of the interplay between mind and body. Compassion allows the exploration to unfold. Wisdom guides the unfolding safely. Medicine is art and science, both of which continue to evolve as society will allow.

SUMMARY POINTS

- Myofascial pain is a regional pain syndrome caused by dysfunction of the nervous system. The pain is based on abnormal physiology, and the expression of the pain is physical.
- Myofascial pain frequently is misdiagnosed as lumbar degenerative disc disease or lumbar herniated disc.
- Routine physical therapy can worsen the symptoms of myofascial pain.
- Myofascial pain frequently coexists with migraine, anxiety, irritable bowel syndrome, and fibromyalgia.
- Successful treatment is based on a multidisciplinary approach, which includes some type of mindful exploration.

CHAPTER 16

Failed-Back Syndrome (Post-Laminectomy Syndrome)

CLINICAL PRESENTATION

Failed-back syndrome, also known as post-laminectomy syndrome, is one of the most frustrating clinical conditions to manage. By definition, patients have undergone at least one surgical treatment for back pain, and very often, patients have undergone multiple lower back surgical procedures. Patients often begin with a laminectomy, followed by lumbar fusion, revision of lumbar fusion, and extension of prior lumbar fusions. Despite the claim by surgeons that each surgery is "perfect," patients become increasingly frustrated and alienated because their pain only worsens over time.

Patients who suffer with failed-back syndrome have essentially constant pain. The pain often is hypersensitive to touch and is burning in nature. The lower back becomes increasingly immobile as patients become increasingly reluctant to challenge their lumbar spine. In addition, the multiple fusions have usually rendered the spine more rigid, and the muscles have developed a hypercontractile state as a response to the multiple interventions.

Pain is usually constant and worsens with any type of prolonged activity, be that sitting, standing, walking, or lying. Pain often awakens the patient from sleep. The patient has usually undergone multiple attempts at physical therapy, only to feel that the therapy worsens the situation. Similarly, he has often undergone multiple attempts at various therapeutic injections, including facet injections and epidural injections, only to obtain no relief or perhaps a worsening of symptoms. In addition to back pain, radiating leg pain may be present, which is similarly constant; this may be burning and hypersensitive to touch. Other neurologic symptoms may be present if the patient previously suffered with nerve compression and nerve injury. There may be a confounding presentation of chronic pain and neurologic symptomatology such as numbness and weakness. Such presentations make it even more difficult to provide a clear-cut clinical diagnosis.

Associated with pain may be a sense of desperation. The patient who undergoes major spinal surgery has a reasonable expectation to improve following surgery. After single or multiple attempts that have led to a sense of surgical failure, the patient comes to believe that nothing can relieve his pain. He also comes to doubt the validity of his symptoms, because he usually is told by surgeons that the spinal canal is perfectly decompressed and the spine is perfectly fused, so there should be no pain. Ultimately, the patient becomes depressed, often with a sense of hopelessness.

CAUSE OF FAILED-BACK SYNDROME

Failed-back syndrome is a neuropathic pain condition, which means that the pain is physiologically mediated and is not caused primarily by an anatomic defect. The transforming event into chronic, neuropathic pain is not clear. In some cases, patients undergo traumatic surgery, with complications thereof, and this becomes the substrate for chronic pain. Others suffered a considerable neurologic damage prior to surgery, and this itself becomes transformed chronic pain from the inciting trauma. Others may have undergone back surgery for relatively uncomplicated reasons, with no complications during surgery, yet they awaken with severe pain, which then becomes transformed into chronic neuropathic pain.

Although several markers may be present, such as overly contracted musculature, hyperirritability of paraspinal muscles, or ongoing injury in lumbar spinal nerves, none of these markers adequately explain the severe constancy of this pain syndrome. It makes more sense to search for a physiological explanation of pain in post-laminectomy syndrome.

Post-thoracotomy pain is severe chest pain that may develop following a thoracotomy, which is the splitting open of the chest bone, usually to perform heart surgery. Post-thoracotomy pain is similar to the pain of post-laminectomy syndrome and is discussed now because of interesting research that has helped clinicians understand the nature of this pain. Such research has not yet been performed for post-laminectomy syndrome.

Although the cause of post-thoracotomy pain is not certain, studies have demonstrated a difference in brain metabolism when comparing thoracotomy patients who have no pain versus those who suffer with post-thoracotomy pain. Post-thoracotomy pain patients—unlike patients who undergo thoracotomy and have no unusual pain postoperatively—develop abnormalities in areas of the emotional brain, such as the cingulate gyrus and prefrontal lobe, even though they had no such abnormalities preoperatively. Thus, some type of reorganization of pain and emotional pathways occurs as a response to the surgery, even though no clear markers or predictors exist for such reorganization. This physiologic reorganization results in chronic, protracted pain.

Physical Examination

The physical examination generally reveals restricted range of motion along all planes of lumbar spinal movement. Generally, multiple areas of tenderness are present in the musculature, and generally, the lumbar scar is well-healed, but may be tender to touch as well. The neurologic examination is unremarkable, unless some complication of nerve damage occurred preoperatively or perioperatively, but this abnormality is not necessarily relevant to the pain syndrome per se.

Imaging and Diagnostic Studies

Other than showing evidence of prior surgery, no specific imaging and diagnostic studies correlate with post-laminectomy syndrome. Those patients who have undergone spinal surgery are more likely than not to have spinal abnormalities, such as degenerative disc changes, and the danger in interpreting imaging studies and trying to provide relevance of such interpretation to the patient is that this may result in recommendations for further surgery.

Electromyography (EMG) and nerve conduction studies may reveal evidence of chronic irritability of lumbar nerves, but should not show any evidence of ongoing, active denervation or irritability.

Some patients with post-laminectomy syndrome do have an anatomic explanation for pain by way of a *pseudoarthrosis*, which means that the spinal fusion is incomplete. In such patients, a single-photon emission computed tomography (SPECT) bone scan will reveal focal abnormalities consistent with a poorly fused lumbar spine. A computed tomography (CT) scan can verify evidence of hardware loosening or pseudoarthrosis by revealing evidence of prolonged, unstable mobility of a spinal segment. When such abnormalities are noted, it then becomes important to differentiate whether these abnormalities are indeed the anatomic basis of the patient's pain or whether they are simply incidental findings. Patients with a true pseudoarthrosis have more situational pain, meaning pain with sudden movement changes, as compared with the more chronic, diffuse pain of failed-back syndrome.

TREATMENT CONSIDERATIONS

Nonsurgical

Patients with failed-back syndrome should undergo multidisciplinary pain management. They are almost universally depressed, with a sense of hopelessness, and are suffering at multiple levels of their being because of chronic pain and failed surgeries. With this in mind, psychological counseling and group therapy should be considered. Such therapy will, at a minimum, help patients to develop better tools of coping with pain. In addition, underlying depression and anxiety can be addressed. Occasionally, mind–body insight leads to other psychological interventions.

Medications generally are required, and combinations of medications often are needed. Antidepressant medication is a cornerstone of treatment. Older, less selective antidepressant medications such as amitriptyline may be used in a low dose to help with sleep deprivation and neuropathic pain. Such medications can be combined with newer-generation antidepressant medications, because these latter medications are more effective in helping to treat depression and anxiety.

Anticonvulsant medications often are utilized and should be chosen according to various patient profiles. As noted previously, some anticonvulsants promote sleep, others promote weight loss, whereas others promote weight gain. Anticonvulsant medications can be used effectively in conjunction with antidepressant medication.

Muscle relaxants may play an important role, because many patients have developed abnormal hypercontractility of the lumbar musculature.

Narcotic analgesics may be required and should be utilized judiciously. Tramadol may be a first-line choice, but sometimes narcotic analgesics that provide more powerful analgesic effects are required. Nonsteroidal anti-inflammatory drugs (NSAIDs) have little role in the chronic treatment of failed-back syndrome.

Manual therapy is an important adjunct, but most patients already have failed numerous attempts at spinal manipulation and physical therapy. Many patients state that they are afraid to undergo physical therapy, because this has only led to an exacerbation of their symptoms.

Spinal manipulation should not be performed, because patients usually have undergone spinal fusion. Physical therapy must focus on myofascial release and craniosacral techniques. Traditional therapy, which includes modalities and routine exercises, usually only exacerbates pain. Acupuncture may play a role, but sometimes the placement of the acupuncture needle leads to an increase in pain, especially in patients who have hypersensitivity to touch in the lumbar region.

Therapeutic injections usually have little role in post-laminectomy syndrome. Most patients already have failed attempts at therapeutic injections prior to surgery and, especially in patients who have undergone spinal fusion, few avenues are left to explore by way of epidural injections, selective nerve root injections, or facet injections.

Surgical

Unless compelling evidence exists of ongoing spinal instability, clear-cut situational pain with pseudoarthrosis, or new evidence of situational pain from nerve root entrapment, further surgical exploration will almost always be a failure. Thus, the clinician must differentiate situational pain from spinal instability or pseudoarthrosis secondary to fusion failure versus the chronic pain of failed-back syndrome.

In patients who have exhausted other aspects of multidisciplinary treatment, a spinal cord stimulator may be useful. Patients must be selected carefully, because many patients may choose to undergo spinal cord stimulator placement with an unrealistic expectation of complete pain relief. Before implanting a permanent stimulator, patients should undergo a stimulator trial and should understand that spinal cord stimulation is again but one aspect of ongoing multidisciplinary pain management. For patients who have responded beneficially to narcotic analgesics but who have developed systemic intolerance, a morphine pump may be considered.

MIND–BODY CONSIDERATIONS

First and foremost, most patients with post-laminectomy syndrome suffer with depression, anxiety, or both. They often have poor coping strategies, and a breakdown in the family and social unit has usually developed as well. Such feelings often are explored and managed quite well in group therapy.

Because failed-back syndrome patients often have a hypersensitivity response, meditation, relaxation, and biofeedback techniques can be of enormous benefit. These avenues allow patients to explore ways to turn inward and gain a sense that they may manage their pain by controlling their body's emotional and physiologic responses.

Patients with post-laminectomy syndrome usually have had a protracted course, and it is sometimes difficult to move patients to the place of their original inciting event. They have been traumatized repeatedly by various therapeutic injections and surgical procedures, and this is a much more prominent aspect of their consciousness than the state of their being when pain first developed. However, as with all pain syndromes, it is useful to explore perceptions at the time of the inciting event, if at all possible, and such exploration should always be done without any presupposed judgments or suggestions.

ILLUSTRATIVE CASE

A 45-year-old man presented to the office with severe, protracted pain in the left lower back region, radiating into the posterior left leg. The patient first injured himself 10 years earlier, when he was pushed down a stairwell, and he developed a herniated lumbar disc. He underwent a single-level laminectomy at L4–L5 for a diagnosis of a herniated lumbar disc at the same level. Prior to surgery, he had low back pain and radiating left leg pain, with associated numbness and a partial foot drop. Although surgery led to resolution of numbness and foot weakness, he had ongoing pain. He described the postoperative pain as burning and constant in nature.

He did not improve with attempts at physical therapy and medication management. He became dependent on narcotic analgesics, although he never utilized more than the prescribed amount of medication. However, his narcotic need escalated rather quickly over a period of 1 year. He underwent two subsequent surgical procedures. Three years following the first surgery, he underwent posterior spinal fusion with placement of instrumentation at L4–L5 and L5–S1. His pain only worsened postoperatively. Again, he described a constant, burning pain, without clear precipitating or palliative features. One year following the second surgery, he underwent revision of the posterior fusion at L4–L5 and L5–S1, and he had extension of fusion by way of an anterior approach (circumferential fusion). Despite the fact that the fusion was apparently "perfect," the pain became increasingly severe.

Over time, the patient was taking high-dose narcotics and becoming increasingly socially isolated. He felt chronically depressed and often harbored passive suicidal thoughts, but never had a concrete plan to kill himself. He had multiple attempts at physical therapy, epidural injections, and trigger-point injections, all to no avail.

The patient's initial physical examination was notable for considerable restriction of trunk range of motion along all planes. He had several areas of tenderness in the lumbar musculature and in the gluteal muscles. His neurologic examination was normal. Imaging studies revealed a solid fusion at L4–L5 and L5–S1, with good decompression and no evidence of spinal derangement otherwise. Electromyography (EMG) and nerve conduction studies showed evidence of chronic left L5 and S1 nerve irritation, without active denervation changes.

The patient was treated in a multidisciplinary manner, which included psychological counseling, group therapy, attempts to change his medication management, and manual physical therapy. He could not be weaned from large doses of various narcotics. He did agree to change his narcotic medication to methadone, in a twice-daily dosage, and he was told that he could only utilize the narcotic medication twice daily. He obtained no benefit from various antidepressant and anticonvulsant medications. In group therapy, he clearly admitted to having been involved in gang activity at the time of the accident, but felt that this was in the past and that the only relevant feature at present was his ongoing pain. He no longer associated with gang activity, and he did not believe that this had any significance to his ongoing symptoms. The patient actively resisted any further attempts at insight-oriented psychotherapy, but he was otherwise a highly compliant individual.

He ultimately was given a trial of spinal cord stimulation, which led to some reduction in his pain. The spinal cord stimulator was then placed permanently and, although he is not pain free, he feels that he can manage his pain better. He continues to take methadone, and he has begun a regular program of exercise. He has come to accept the fact that, although his pain is reduced by no more than 50% from when he first began treatment, he at least feels that his coping strategies are better. He also has agreed to try to explore alternative career opportunities.

Author's Note

This patient represents the highly complex nature of failed-back syndrome. In this particular case, the patient underwent repeated attempts of spinal fusion, despite the absence of any clear-cut indications for such treatment. Spinal fusion is indicated in patients who have spinal instability or who are at risk of developing spinal instability. This patient had neither, and the fusion was simply performed because he had ongoing complaints of pain following a laminectomy. This is a trap into which too many spinal surgeons and patients fall.

Although this patient may have a significant, somewhat dissociated posttraumatic stress component to his persona, he is either not willing or is not capable of exploring this, and such exploration cannot be forced on an individual. By definition, multidisciplinary pain management means that all avenues can be explored, and the avenue that makes the most sense for the individual patient should be pursued further. In this case, spinal cord stimulator made sense, and the patient did obtain some improvement from this intervention.

SUMMARY POINTS

■ Failed-back syndrome is a neuropathic pain condition and is not the result of an ongoing anatomic problem in the spine.

■ Patients with failed-back syndrome usually have coexisting depression, and may withdraw considerably from family and society.

■ Treatment should be multidisciplinary, including psychological and group counseling when possible.

■ Further surgery usually worsens this problem. Spinal cord stimulator may be appropriate in select cases.

CHAPTER 17

Chronic Pain Syndrome

CLINICAL PRESENTATION

In chronic pain syndrome, a patient has pain that has persisted months or years longer than one might expect from an inciting event. Several maladaptive features are associated with the pain. In patients with chronic pain syndrome, suffering occurs at every level of being: physical, emotional, mental, social, and spiritual. In essence, the patient becomes defined by pain rather than by a more soulful sense of self. Chronic pain syndrome may be seen as a combination of any of the other clinical syndromes discussed previously. Chronic pain syndrome may be one of the most challenging clinical syndromes for clinicians to address and manage.

Chronic pain syndrome entails chronic neuropathic pain and, as such, represents a dysfunction of the nervous system. There is no clear consensus as to why patients develop chronic pain syndrome. What is clear is that an inciting event or events occur, and patients seemingly never recover. Rather, pain persists, takes on a life of its own, and the patient becomes imprisoned, living a life of pain every waking moment.

Chronic pain syndrome can develop in any region of the body. Some patients have chronic, refractory headache. Others have chronic, refractory neck pain. Others have unrelenting low back pain. Others have more diffuse body and joint pain. Chronic pain syndrome is distinguished from the chronic pain that occurs as a result of inflammatory or mechanical causes by the fact that no situational fluctuations to the pain occur. Chronic pain syndrome is essentially indistinguishable from post-laminectomy syndrome if the patient has undergone lumbar spine surgery.

Patients who have chronic pain syndrome in the region of the lower back typically have pain that never ceases. Patients have difficulty sleeping at night because of pain. Pain may be described as sharp, burning, electric, shock-like, lancinating, achy, or simply as a diffuse, deep-seated pain. Sensitivity to touch may be present in the region of the pain.

Sometimes, associated autonomic features are present, in that there may be alterations in skin color or temperature and even regional changes in the hair growth pattern. Because of musculoskeletal disuse, bone loss may develop. In addition, muscle contractures and even bony contractures can occur. In women of childbearing age with chronic pain syndrome, menstrual irregularity is common.

Patients generally complain that pain worsens with any type of prolonged activity, and pain also is present at rest. Weather fluctuations may influence pain, and day-to-day emotional fluctuations may precipitate pain. Typically, patients have undergone numerous therapeutic interventions, including epidural injections, facet blocks, surgical procedures, multiple trials of medications, and multiple trials of physical therapy and spinal manipulation.

Depression is the rule in patients with chronic pain syndrome. Often, patients have a *flat affect*, which means that they no longer express a range of emotions when speaking. Many patients have lost a sense of hope. Relationships have become defined by pain, and the family unit often is dysfunctional because the patient suffering with pain can no longer become meaningfully engaged in family or social relationships. Very often, patients are out of work and receiving disability compensation.

Patients often feel desperate, and they may have sought a multitude of alternative treatment strategies. Too often, patients have been taken advantage of by clinicians who offer unrealistic hope. Many patients with chronic pain syndrome seem to be going through the motions when they are undergoing an evaluation by a clinician, because they feel that they are not being heard; very often, they think that no one believes them. This is not surprising given the fact that multiple treatments have failed and, very often, clinicians will simply say that no adequate explanation exists for the patient's pain, thus suggesting that the pain must have a psychosomatic origin.

CAUSE OF CHRONIC PAIN SYNDROME

The cause of chronic pain lies within nervous system dysfunction. A concept in neuroscience called *brain plasticity* means that the brain can reorganize following an insult to the body or nervous system. There is no question that brain reorganization occurs in chronic pain patients, but the reorganization is not necessarily because of a lesion in the nervous system. Rather, the reorganization occurs as a result of a multitude of physical and emotional responses to a major inciting event or multiple inciting events.

Genetic factors may predispose to the development of chronic pain syndrome. Some studies suggest genetic alterations in pain receptors of the spinal cord, and these alterations predispose such patients to neuropathic pain. Other evidence suggests that patients who have suffered prior trauma or abuse are more predisposed to developing chronic pain syndrome when compared with the general population. This latter explanation should not lead physicians to presume that patients with chronic pain syndrome have been prior victims of abuse.

Even in patients who suffer with chronic pain syndrome, fluctuations in pain may occur that have an anatomic basis. Thus, clinicians must always be aware of this possibility. For example, a patient suffering with chronic pain syndrome may develop a superimposed lumbar disc herniation, a severe strain in the iliopsoas muscle, or an acute spinal fracture, all as a result of prior, chronic maladaptations. Any one of a number of possibilities of more acute, anatomically based pain is possible in patients who suffer with chronic pain. Addressing these factors is key, while keeping in mind that they are only one part of the larger cycle of pain.

PHYSICAL EXAMINATION

No classic physical examination findings are present in patients who suffer with chronic pain. More often than not, several maladaptive musculoskeletal findings are evident when performing a careful physical examination. This may include abnormal movements of the lumbar spine in flexion and extension, abnormal contractility of supporting lumbar spine musculature, or chronic spasm and sensitivity of muscles, which can be noted by palpation. The neurologic exam is unremarkable unless the chronic pain syndrome has developed in the setting of a prior neurologic insult, for example, a nerve root injury as part of a lumbar spine disorder.

IMAGING AND DIAGNOSTIC STUDIES

No classic imaging and diagnostic studies are definitive in patients who suffer with chronic pain syndrome. Some evidence may be present of prior surgical interventions and, as with patients who suffer with failed-back syndrome, incidental findings of degenerative disc changes or chronic disc herniations may be noted. Electromyography (EMG) and nerve conduction studies may show evidence of chronic lumbar nerve root irritation, but do not reveal meaningful active denervation changes. Very often, patients are subjected to a multitude of imaging and diagnostic studies, including but not limited to multiple plain radiographs, multiple magnetic resonance imaging (MRI) studies, routine and triple phase bone scan studies, EMG and nerve conduction studies, myelogram, and detailed rheumatologic evaluation. None of these studies provides a compelling explanation for the patient's pain.

In functional brain imaging studies, such as functional brain MRI or positron emission tomography (PET) scanning, patients who suffer with chronic pain syndrome may demonstrate abnormal metabolism and hyper-responsiveness in several areas of the *limbic brain*, which is the largely nonconscious, emotional brain. These studies demonstrate that the simplistic view of pain pathways no longer holds for patients with chronic pain syndrome.

TREATMENT CONSIDERATIONS

Nonsurgical

Patients with chronic pain syndrome benefit from psychological counseling. However, the manner in which this is presented to the patient is important. Patients should not be led to believe that they are undergoing psychological counseling because their pain is psychogenic in origin. Rather, patients require psychological counseling because an almost universal, coexisting depression and sense of hopelessness are present. Coping strategies are usually poor, and the family unit often has broken down. Individual psychological counseling in conjunction with group therapy is extremely beneficial.

Medication management usually includes a combination approach. Because patients frequently have a disruption of their sleep cycle, medications such as amitriptyline (an early-generation antidepressant medication) or an anticonvulsant with sedative properties can be useful to help restore sleep. Low-dose amitriptyline may have pain-relieving properties in and of itself. Similarly, anticonvulsants should be titrated upward, as tolerated and needed, because they may provide an important avenue of pain relief.

Newer-generation antidepressants also may play an important role in helping to treat depression and anxiety. Narcotic analgesics may be an important part of treatment, because anything that leads to pain reduction may help to improve quality of life. Muscle relaxants also may play an important role in patients who have chronic, hypercontracted musculature. Nonsteroidal anti-inflammatory drugs (NSAIDs) have little role in the long-term management of chronic pain syndrome.

Manual therapy plays an extremely important role. However, such therapy must be performed with a long-term vision in mind. Most patients have already been through multiple attempts at physical therapy or chiropractic care. Manual therapy should be performed with a focus on myofascial release and craniosacral technique, in an attempt to help the patient turn inward, become more attuned to his body, and to gradually help restore proper posture in body mechanics.

Therapeutic injections may or may not play a role, depending on the clinical manifestation at hand. Some patients who suffer with chronic pain syndrome also have situational, mechanical pain. For example, some patients with chronic low back pain also develop more specific facet jamming; such patients may obtain some relief from facet injections. However, if such injections are utilized, it should be understood that they are not the answer, but only a small part of the multidisciplinary treatment. If patients obtain meaningful benefit, then a facet rhizotomy procedure should be considered. Usually, epidural corticosteroid injections or selective nerve root injections are ineffective.

Once patients have developed some aspects of pain control and coping strategies, a gentle exercise program should be encouraged. This should be coordinated carefully with the physical therapist.

Surgical

One must proceed very cautiously with any thoughts of surgery in patients who suffer with chronic pain syndrome. Patients are often desperate, and even physicians can be desperate to try to cure the patient of his malady. It is important to remember that chronic pain syndrome represents a dysfunction of the nervous system, and surgical interventions to correct anatomic lesions or deficits may only lead to an augmented pain response postoperatively. Unless a clearly defined, anatomically well-localized cause of one aspect of the patient's chronic pain syndrome exists, all surgical considerations should be avoided. Physicians should explain to patients that surgery may only worsen the situation.

In cases of well-localized pain, spinal cord stimulator may be considered as part of a well-disciplined, multidisciplinary treatment. Again, the lure may be that spinal cord stimulator will alleviate the patient's problem; this is unlikely in patients who have chronic pain syndrome. If spinal cord stimulator can help to alleviate some pain, and if patients can achieve better coping strategies and obtain a better sense of pain relief with medication management and manual interventions, then such an intervention can be considered.

In patients who clearly benefit from narcotic analgesics, but who cannot tolerate systemic side effects, then a morphine pump may be considered. As with a spinal cord stimulator, this should be part of a multidisciplinary approach, not a unilateral intervention.

MIND–BODY CONSIDERATIONS

Mind–body considerations play a pivotal role in managing patients with chronic pain syndrome. Such a patient has been suffering considerably, usually with a marked dissociation between the patient's emotions and his sense of physical pain. Initial mind–body approaches should include meditation and relaxation exercises, possibly coupled with biofeedback or similar strategies. At a minimum, such strategies should help the patient cope and gain a sense of control over his own physiology and pain responses. Sometimes, such interventions open the door to greater mind–body insights.

The one potential trap of mind–body therapy in treating patients with chronic pain syndrome is the assumption that the patient is hiding something from his past. This is a dangerous assumption in which a patient is led to believe that he is the cause of his problem. Although we can assume that depression, anxiety, and pain intermix with chronic pain syndrome, we cannot presume that depression or prior psychological factors are the sole cause of chronic pain syndrome.

ILLUSTRATIVE CASE

A 25-year-old woman presented to the office with complaints of chronic low back pain of 10 years' duration. The patient first recalls developing low back pain when she was at soccer camp. She suffered a fall during training and felt a pop in her lower back. She had considerable pain and asked to be removed from soccer practice. Because this was a sleep-away camp, a decision had to be made as to whether the patient could remain at camp. When her parents received a phone call from the camp counselor, they were insistent that the patient remain at camp. The patient was distraught over this decision, because she did not believe that she was capable of participating meaningfully in soccer training.

The athletic trainer on site agreed to try to work with the patient. From the patient's perspective, the athletic trainer was cold hearted and mean spirited. He told the patient that the pain was imaginary and that she simply was not strong-willed enough to continue in camp. He forced her to do certain exercises against her will and told the patient that she was to say nothing to family members or other camp counselors. She felt threatened by the athletic trainer and did not divulge this information until years later.

When the patient returned home from camp, her pain was severe. The pain was located in the midline lower back, with some radiating pain into the left leg. An orthopedic surgeon ultimately diagnosed a herniated lumbar disc and recommended physical therapy. She did not improve with physical therapy, and her condition only seemed to worsen. Ultimately, at age 16, she underwent a lumbar laminectomy. Postoperatively, the pain became severe, with an increase in pain in the left leg. The pain in the leg became inordinately severe; the leg became swollen, discolored, and hypersensitive to touch.

The patient then was diagnosed with *reflex sympathetic dystrophy (complex regional pain syndrome)*, a syndrome in which the autonomic nervous system becomes overactive in response to tissue injury and intertwines with the normal pain pathways. The patient underwent a series of therapeutic injections directed at treating the reflex sympathetic dystrophy. Although the leg pain subsided somewhat, she had persistent low back and leg pain that was otherwise unresponsive to physical therapy and medical management.

At age 18, the patient underwent spinal fusion at the L4–L5 level. This only led to a marked worsening of her pain. Although she no longer had active reflex sympathetic dystrophy in her left leg, she developed an essentially constant low back and radiating left leg pain, unresponsive to all interventions, which worsened with all physical activity. The patient had essentially abandoned all forms of exercise. She gained 50 pounds. She began performing poorly academically, and she withdrew from her friends. She finished high school but did not feel capable of going to college. She has since been working part-time, performing clerical work.

Her physical examination demonstrated a marked hesitation by the patient to attempt even limited spine range of motion. Some avoidance behavior was present as well, in that the patient preferred not to have her left leg touched. No abnormal skin color or temperature changes in the leg were noted, and the leg was not swollen. The neurologic examination was normal.

Imaging and diagnostic studies revealed a solid fusion at the L4–L5 level. A single-photon emission computed tomography (SPECT) bone scan was normal. Electromyography (EMG) and nerve conduction studies were normal. The rheumatologic workup was negative.

The patient began treatment with psychotherapy, group therapy, manual physical therapy, and a combination of anticonvulsant and antidepressant medication. For over 1 year, the patient's pain did not improve, and she required larger doses of narcotic analgesics. At one point, she was receiving a 100 μg fentanyl patch every 2 days in conjunction with gabapentin, carisoprodol, venlafaxine, and trazadone. She seemed to develop an increasing sense of despondency and required psychiatric hospitalization because of a suicide attempt.

In addition to group therapy, psychotherapy, physical therapy, and medication management, the patient underwent massage therapy with a focus on intuitive manual techniques. During one session, the patient became inconsolable, developing repeated flashbacks of having been sexually abused by her uncle between the ages of 7 and 10. The uncle had acted as the patient's baby-sitter over a period of 3 years, and he had the complete trust of other members of the family unit. The uncle not only sexually abused the patient, but also intimidated her, threatened her, and at one point, had injured her back during an abusive act. He told the patient that she was never to tell anyone about this incident, otherwise there would be serious repercussions to the entire family.

With these flashbacks, the patient became psychiatrically unstable, requiring intense psychiatric intervention. This prompted two additional psychiatric hospitalizations. As she ultimately became more psychiatrically stable, she returned to the massage therapist and also continued with group therapy, psychotherapy, and manual physical therapy. She gained a sense of confidence in trying to integrate her various emotions, and she came to understand the possible linkage between the development of low back pain at the soccer camp, the psychological abuse she received from the athletic trainer, and her prior history of abuse.

As she came to reconcile these various emotions, she also developed the courage to report her uncle's actions to her family members. Although initially incredulous, over time the family members embraced the patient's story, and a more healing environment developed. Over the long term, the patient has improved considerably. She has a much deeper sense of feeling validated. She has much better coping strategies, her pain has diminished considerably, and she has enrolled in college part-time.

Author's Note

This case should not be interpreted simplistically. It is by no means meant to be an indication that patients with chronic pain have suffered prior abuse. However, this case does illustrate that such stories occur, and unfortunately, such stories are not uncommon. This is in keeping with the medical literature and with the author's personal experience. The other notable feature of the story is that the patient's flashbacks led to the possibility for a healing journey to take place. Had suggestions been delivered to the patient that she must be a victim of abuse, this could have had catastrophic consequences.

Ultimately, this story demonstrates the potential redemptive value of wholistic multidisciplinary pain medicine. While trying to help patients in alleviating pain, we can be aware that at any point in time, a patient may become ready to change the course of treatment, or circumstances may change that dictate a change in treatment.

Patients with chronic pain often build protective walls around themselves. They suffer tremendously, and they may have been let down by loved ones and by society. In working with such patients in a nonjudgmental and compassionate way, while maintaining good clinical judgment, glimpses of stories may evolve that hold the key to solving a complex puzzle. As the puzzle is pieced together, the patient and treating clinicians come to understand they are taking a journey—a healing journey—that can be measured best in terms of grace-filled moments.

SUMMARY POINTS

- Chronic pain syndrome can develop from any one of a number of clinical syndromes. In essence, every aspect of the patient becomes defined by pain.
- Patients with chronic pain syndrome are universally depressed, and a high incidence of breakdown in the family and social structure is present.
- Functional brain imaging studies of patients with chronic pain syndrome may reveal abnormalities in parts of the brain that mediate nonconscious emotions.
- There may be genetic predispositions to chronic pain syndrome, and there may also be a history of prior personal, emotional, or physical abuse. However, many patients have neither of these predispositions, and such predispositions should never be assumed.
- Treatment for chronic pain syndrome should be multidisciplinary, including individual and group psychological counseling when possible.
- Treatment should be long term; at any point in time, the treatment may change considerably, based on patient–clinician results and experiences.

CHAPTER 18

Closing Thoughts

I wonder if the medicine man from the Ivory Coast would understand this book? Indeed, I wonder if this book makes sense to many readers, patients and treating clinicians alike? In our society, we are inundated with quick-fix solutions, ranging from curative surgical techniques to wonderful medications that are advertised during our favorite television programs. Any astute observer who cares to take a step back would understand that quick fixes, especially for low back pain, do not always work.

As a physician, I am saddened to realize how many people suffer with chronic or recurring low back pain. As a compassionate human being, my heart aches when I realize that chronic low back pain is so often mismanaged with false hope and false expectation. As a scientist, I shudder to realize that so little understanding exists for the physiology, anatomy, and management of chronic pain by the multitude of clinicians who claim to offer certain remedies.

This book is by no means definitive. Indeed, it serves as an introduction to a vast problem, and my hope is that the reader will come to understand that many doors may need to be opened before the proper path of treatment begins. Where to turn? There is no easy answer. Sometimes it is word of mouth. Sometimes it is finding a good resource. Sometimes it is trial and error. I truly hope this book may become one resource for beginning a journey to understanding, managing, and working in a healing manner with the low back—as part of our being.

Glossary of Terms

Acetaminophen   An over-the-counter pain medication that is not in the class of nonsteroidal anti-inflammatory drugs.

Actiq   The brand name for transmucosal fentanyl, formulated as a short-acting narcotic analgesic medication.

Acupuncture   A Chinese medical treatment in which needles are placed in various points of the body for the purpose of balancing *chi* energy.

Acute pain   Pain that develops immediately after an inciting or noxious event.

Aleve   Brand name for over-the-counter naproxen, a nonsteroidal anti-inflammatory drug.

Amitriptyline   A tricyclic antidepressant medication that often is used to treat neuropathic pain.

Anabolic steroid   A class of medication that enhances muscle strength and prevents tissue breakdown after heavy muscular exertion.

Analgesic   Any medication that provides pain relief.

Anaprox   Brand name for prescription-strength naproxen sodium, a nonsteroidal anti-inflammatory drug.

Anesthesiologist   A physician who specializes in providing anesthesia to patients. An anesthesiologist may subspecialize in pain medicine.

Anticoagulant   A medication that thins the blood, thereby increasing the risk of bleeding.

Antidepressant   A class of medication utilized to treat depression.

Antihistamine	A class of medication utilized to treat allergies and allergic reactions.
Atrophy	Wasting or shrinkage of muscle size, either from disuse or from an underlying disease process.
Autoimmune	A reaction of the immune system in which part of the individual's body is attacked by its own immune system.
Avinza	Brand name for long-acting morphine, a narcotic analgesic medication.
Baclofen	A medication utilized to treat spasticity and muscle spasm.
Benadryl	Brand name for over-the-counter diphenhydramine, an antihistamine medication.
Bextra	Brand name for valdecoxib, a COX-2 nonsteroidal anti-inflammatory drug that has been removed from the market.
Biofeedback	A technique in which the patient learns various relaxation techniques by receiving immediate computer feedback regarding muscle tone or skin temperature.
Bone scan	An imaging study that assesses the health of the bones following the injection of a radioisotope into the veins.
Bupropion	An antidepressant medication that blocks the reuptake of dopamine and norepinephrine.
Carbamazepine	An anticonvulsant medication that is also utilized to treat neuropathic pain.
Carisoprodol	A muscle relaxant medication.
Celebrex	Brand name for celecoxib, a COX-2 nonsteroidal anti-inflammatory drug.
Celecoxib	A COX-2 nonsteroidal anti-inflammatory drug.
Celexa	Brand name for citalopram, a serotonin specific reuptake inhibitor antidepressant medication.
Cerebral palsy	A neurologic condition that develops as a result of a brain insult to the developing child *in utero* or at birth. Patients frequently present with spasticity.

212

Chlorzoxazone	A muscle relaxant medication.
Chronic pain	Pain that persists at least one month longer than one might reasonably expect following an inciting or noxious event.
Chronic pain syndrome	A medical condition characterized by chronic pain and maladaptation socially, psychologically, and physically.
Chiropractor	A nonphysician doctor who specializes in spinal manipulation.
Citalopram	A serotonin specific reuptake inhibitor antidepressant medication.
Combunox	Brand name for a combination of ibuprofen and short-acting oxycodone, which is a narcotic analgesic medication.
Computed tomography scan (CT scan)	A computerized x-ray machine that provides three-dimensional images of the body.
Corticosteroid	A potent anti-inflammatory medication.
Coumadin	Brand name for warfarin, an anticoagulant medication.
COX enzyme	The enzyme system that is divided into COX-1 or COX-2 in nonsteroidal anti-inflammatory drugs. The COX-1 medications prolong bleeding time and are more prone to cause gastric irritation, as opposed to COX-2 medications, which do not prolong bleeding time and cause relatively less gastric irritation.
Cyclobenzaprine	A muscle relaxant medication.
Cymbalta	Brand name for duloxetine, a serotonin-norepinephrine reuptake inhibitor antidepressant medication.
Darvocet	Brand name for a combination of acetaminophen and propoxyphene, which is a short-acting narcotic analgesic medication.
Darvon	Brand name for propoxyphene, a short-acting narcotic analgesic medication.

Delirium	A mental state characterized by confusion and agitation, usually in association with a medical illness or from drug intoxication.
Depakene	Brand name for valproic acid, an anticonvulsant medication.
Depakote	Brand name for valproic acid, an anticonvulsant medication.
Desipramine	A tricyclic antidepressant medication.
Desyrel	Brand name for trazodone, an older antidepressant medication commonly utilized to treat insomnia.
Diazepam	A sedating medication commonly used to treat spasticity, muscle spasm, and anxiety.
Diclofenac	A nonsteroidal anti-inflammatory drug.
Diflunisal	A nonsteroidal anti-inflammatory drug.
Dilaudid	Brand name for hydromorphone, a short-acting narcotic analgesic medication.
Diphenhydramine	An over-the-counter antihistamine medication commonly used to treat allergies and allergic reactions.
Dolobid	Brand name for diflunisal, a nonsteroidal anti-inflammatory drug.
Dopamine	A brain neurochemical that is involved in the experience of ecstasy and that also mediates certain aspects of motor control.
Discogram	A diagnostic procedure performed by a radiologist or pain medicine specialist in which dye is injected directly into the lumbar disc for the purpose of both analyzing the pain response and imaging the disc.
Duloxetine	A serotonin-norepinephrine reuptake inhibitor antidepressant medication.
Duragesic	Brand name for a transdermal preparation of fentanyl, a narcotic analgesic. This preparation is slowly absorbed through the skin over 3 days.
Effexor	Brand name for venlafaxine, a serotonin-norepinephrine reuptake inhibitor antidepressant medication.

Elavil	Brand name for amitriptyline, a tricyclic antidepressant medication.
Electromyography (EMG)/nerve conduction studies	A test in which the nerves and muscles are examined to assess whether nerve or muscle dysfunction is present. The nerves are stimulated by an electric shock, and the muscles are tested via needle insertion through the skin. A specialized machine provides the information, which is interpreted by a physician specially trained for this procedure.
Endocet	Brand name for a combination of acetaminophen and oxycodone, which is a short-acting narcotic analgesic medication.
Endodan	Brand name for a combination of aspirin and oxycodone, which is a short-acting narcotic analgesic medication.
Epilepsy	A neurologic condition characterized by repeated seizures. Most patients with epilepsy require treatment with an anticonvulsant medication.
Erector spinae muscles	Superficial muscles in the back that allow for trunk extension.
Etiology	A medical term that refers to causation.
Etodolac	A nonsteroidal anti-inflammatory drug.
Facet	The part of the bony spine that allows for smooth, gliding movements of the trunk.
Facet joint	A complex of two facets that normally works in a smooth, contiguous manner to allow for trunk movement.
Failed-back surgery	Terminology that means a patient has undergone spine surgery, yet has ongoing pain that requires medical treatment.
Family medicine physician	A physician who is a generalist.
Fentanyl	A narcotic analgesic that may be prepared as a short-acting transmucosal or long-acting transdermal preparation, or which may be given intravenously.

Flexeril	Brand name for cyclobenzaprine, a muscle relaxant medication.
Fluoxetine	The first of the newer-generation antidepressant medications that are called serotonin specific reuptake inhibitors.
Gabapentin	An anticonvulsant medication commonly utilized to treat neuropathic pain.
Gamma-amino butyric acid (GABA)	A brain neurochemical that mediates various neurologic manifestations, including spasticity and seizures.
Glucocortico-steroid	Another name for corticosteroid, a powerful anti-inflammatory medication.
Glutamate	A brain neurochemical that has excitatory and sometimes damaging properties.
Gout	A medical condition characterized by periodic painful inflammation of the large toe.
Hydrocodone	A short-acting narcotic analgesic medication.
Hydromorphone	A short-acting narcotic analgesic medication.
Iliopsoas muscle	A muscle that connects the low back to the leg and allows for hip flexion.
Imipramine	A tricyclic antidepressant medication.
Indocin	Brand name for indomethacin, a powerful non-steroidal anti-inflammatory drug.
Indomethacin	A powerful nonsteroidal anti-inflammatory drug.
Integrative medicine	Integrative medicine refers to the practice of combining conventional medicine with complementary and alternative medicine. Integrative medicine may be used interchangeably with "wholistic medicine."
Internist	A physician who specializes in the general practice of internal medicine.
Intrathecal	The space around the spine that is filled with spinal fluid. Medications may be delivered into the intrathecal space.

Intravenous	Into the vein.
Kadian	Brand name for long-acting morphine, a narcotic analgesic medication.
Ketorolac	A nonsteroidal anti-inflammatory drug.
Lamictal	Brand name for lamotrigine, an anticonvulsant medication.
Lamotrigine	An anticonvulsant medication that also is used to treat neuropathic pain.
Lesion	A medical term that refers to any structural abnormality in the body.
Lidocaine	An anesthetic that is commonly used by dentists before performing painful procedures. Lidocaine may be delivered transdermally as a patch to treat localized areas of pain in the body.
Lidoderm patch	Brand name for a transdermal preparation of lidocaine.
Lioresal	Brand name for baclofen, a medication that treats spasticity and that may be used as a muscle relaxant.
Lodine	Brand name for etodolac, a nonsteroidal anti-inflammatory drug.
Lorcet	Brand name for a combination of acetaminophen and hydrocodone, which is a short-acting narcotic analgesic medication.
Lortab	Brand name for a combination of acetaminophen and hydrocodone, which is a short-acting narcotic analgesic medication.
Lumbar disc	The cushioning and stabilizing connection between two lumbar vertebrae.
Lyrica	Brand name for pregabalin, an anticonvulsant medication commonly utilized to treat neuropathic pain.
Magnetic resonance imaging (MRI)	A computerized machine that provides detailed three-dimensional images of the body by utilizing magnetic energy.

Massage therapist A clinician who is trained in massage therapy.

Meloxicam A nonsteroidal anti-inflammatory drug.

Metaxalone A muscle relaxant medication.

Methadone A long-acting narcotic analgesic medication that also binds to non-narcotic brain and spinal cord receptors.

Methocarbamol A muscle relaxant medication.

Mirtazapine A sedating antidepressant medication that interacts with serotonin and norepinephrine pathways.

Mobic Brand name for meloxicam, a nonsteroidal anti-inflammatory drug.

Morphine A narcotic analgesic medication; it is the standard to which other narcotic analgesics are measured.

MS Contin Brand name for long-acting morphine, a narcotic analgesic medication.

MSIR Brand name for short-acting morphine, a narcotic analgesic medication.

Multifidus muscle One of the deep muscles of the back that allows for trunk rotation and extension.

Multiple sclerosis An autoimmune medical condition in which the immune system attacks the covering of nerves, leading to neurologic difficulties such as weakness and loss of balance.

Muscle fibers The small layers of muscle within a large muscle.

Myelogram A procedure in which dye is placed within the spinal canal for the purpose of obtaining a detailed image of the spine.

Myofascial pain Pain that develops within a region of the body from a physiologic imbalance and not from localized inflammation.

Nabumetone A nonsteroidal anti-inflammatory drug.

Naprosyn Brand name for naproxen, a nonsteroidal anti-inflammatory drug.

Naproxen A nonsteroidal anti-inflammatory drug that may be obtained over-the-counter or as a prescription.

Narcotic analgesic	A class of medication that is the most powerful of the pain-relieving medications.
Neurologist	A physician who specializes in diagnosing and managing diseases of the brain, spinal cord, and nerves.
Neurontin	Brand name for gabapentin, an anticonvulsant medication.
Neuropathic pain	Pain that is caused by a lesion or dysfunction of the nervous system.
Neurosurgeon	A physician who specializes in treating diseases of the brain, spinal cord, and nerves through surgery.
NMDA receptor	A brain and spinal cord receptor that influences the physiology of pain signals.
Nociceptive pain	Pain that is generated by activation of nerve fibers following nerve irritation from a mechanical, chemical, or thermal stimulus.
Nociceptors	Nerve receptors that are responsible for sending pain signals following nerve irritation from a mechanical, chemical, or thermal stimulus.
Norco	Brand name for a combination of acetaminophen and hydrocodone, which is a short-acting narcotic analgesic medication.
Norepinephrine	A brain neurochemical that mediates many responses, including mood and pain.
Norflex	Brand name for orphenadrine, a muscle relaxant medication.
Norgesic	Brand name for a combination of aspirin and orphenadrine, which is a muscle relaxant medication.
Norpramin	Brand name for desipramine, a tricyclic antidepressant medication.
Nortriptyline	A tricyclic antidepressant medication.
Opioid	Pertaining to the opioid system, which is the body's innate narcotic-like pathways.
Oramorph	Brand name for a liquid formulation of short-acting morphine, a narcotic analgesic medication.

Orphenadrine	A muscle relaxant medication.
Orthopedic surgeon	A physician who specializes in surgery of the skeletal system.
Osteopathic doctor	A physician who has completed an accredited program of study in an osteopathic medical school, which is a medical school that focuses on the spine more so than traditional medical schools.
Osteophytes	Calcium spurs that develop in the spine as a result of degenerative changes in the intervertebral discs.
Oxcarbazepine	An anticonvulsant medication.
Oxycodone	A narcotic analgesic that may be prepared as a short- or long-acting medication, alone or in combination with other drugs.
OxyContin	Brand name for long-acting oxycodone, a narcotic analgesic medication.
Pain center	A multidisciplinary treatment facility devoted to managing patients with chronic pain.
Pain medicine	A branch of medicine devoted to the diagnosis and management of patients with pain syndromes.
Pamelor	Brand name for nortriptyline, a tricyclic antidepressant medication.
Paraflex	Brand name for chlorzoxazone, a muscle relaxant medication.
Parafon forte	Brand name for chlorzoxazone, a muscle relaxant medication.
Paroxetine	A serotonin specific reuptake inhibitor antidepressant medication.
Paxil	Brand name for paroxetine, a serotonin specific reuptake inhibitor antidepressant medication.
Percocet	Brand name for a combination of acetaminophen and short-acting oxycodone, which is a narcotic analgesic medication.

Percodan	Brand name for a combination of aspirin and short-acting oxycodone, which is a narcotic analgesic medication.
Physiatrist	A physician who specializes in musculoskeletal rehabilitation medicine.
Physical therapist	A nonphysician clinician who specializes in rehabilitation, using a combination of modalities, hands-on treatment, and exercise protocols.
Physician	A medical doctor who has completed an accredited medical school or school of osteopathic medicine, and who may practice medicine as a medical doctor.
Platelets	Blood elements that are responsible for the first line of defense in preventing bleeding following tissue trauma.
Pregabalin	An anticonvulsant medication commonly used to treat neuropathic pain.
Propoxyphene	A short-acting narcotic analgesic medication.
Prostaglandin	A group of blood elements that are involved in diverse pathways, including inflammation. Nonsteroidal anti-inflammatory drugs work in part by inhibiting the prostaglandin pathway.
Prostate	A male gland just below the neck of the bladder. Prostate enlargement leads to urinary retention in men.
Prototypic	Pertaining to the original or model form.
Prozac	Brand name for fluoxetine, which is the original serotonin specific reuptake inhibitor antidepressant medication.
Psychiatrist	A physician who specializes in treating psychiatric medical conditions.
Psychologist	A nonphysician clinician who specializes in diagnosing and managing psychological conditions.
Psychosomatic	Terminology that refers to physical symptoms that are caused from emotional imbalance.

Quadratus lumborum	One of the deep rotator muscles of the spine that permits trunk rotation and extension.
Radiologist	A physician who specializes in performing and interpreting imaging studies of the body and the brain.
Receptor	A specific chemical–physical attachment to a cell that becomes activated by a matching chemical or protein, which then leads to a cell reaction.
Reflexologist	A nonphysician clinician who specializes in treating various points in the feet that correspond to purported *chi* energy pathways.
Relafen	Brand name for nabumetone, a nonsteroidal anti-inflammatory drug.
Remeron	Brand name for mirtazapine, an antidepressant medication that is sedating and affects the norepinephrine and serotonin pathways.
Rheumatologist	A physician who specializes in the diagnosis and management of degenerative, inflammatory, and autoimmune musculoskeletal disorders.
Robaxin	Brand name for methocarbamol, a muscle relaxant medication.
Robaxisal	Brand name for a combination of aspirin and methocarbamol, which is a muscle relaxant medication.
Rofecoxib	A COX-2 nonsteroidal anti-inflammatory drug that has been removed from the market.
Roxicet	Brand name for a combination of acetaminophen and short-acting oxycodone, which is a narcotic analgesic medication.
Sciatica	A condition characterized by pain that radiates from the low back region into the back and side of the leg as a result of irritation of the sciatic nerve.
Sciatic nerve	A large nerve that is formed from the joining together of several nerves from the lumbo-sacral spine.
Seizure	A medical condition that is caused by abnormal brain electrical excitation. Seizure types may range from

mild changes in behavior to violent shaking of the body with unconsciousness.

Selective serotonin reuptake inhibitor A group of antidepressant medications that make serotonin more available by preventing its normal re-entry into the cell.

Serotonin A brain neurochemical that influences various manifestations, including depression and pain.

Serotonin-norepinephrine reuptake inhibitor A group of antidepressant medications that make serotonin and norepinephrine more available by preventing their normal re-entry into the cell.

Sertraline A serotonin specific reuptake inhibitor antidepressant medication.

Skelaxin Brand name for metaxalone, a muscle relaxant medication.

Soma Brand name for carisoprodol, a muscle relaxant medication.

Spasticity A manifestation of a neurologic condition characterized by increased muscle tone, muscle stiffness, and reduction in fine motor movement.

Subcutaneous Just under the skin.

Tegretol Brand name for carbamazepine, an anticonvulsant medication.

Tizanidine A medication that reduces spasticity and acts as a muscle relaxant.

Tofranil Brand name for imipramine, a tricyclic antidepressant medication.

Tolerance A term that indicates a habituation response to the effects of narcotic analgesics.

Topamax Brand name for topiramate, an anticonvulsant medication.

Topiramate An anticonvulsant medication that is also commonly utilized to treat neuropathic pain and headache.

Toradol A nonsteroidal anti-inflammatory drug that may be given orally, intravenously, or intramuscularly.

Tramadol	A short-acting narcotic-like analgesic medication.
Transdermal	Application of medication or other substance via a skin patch.
Transmucosal	Application of medication or other substance through the mucous membrane, usually through the cheeks inside the mouth.
Trazodone	An older antidepressant medication that is often used to treat insomnia.
Tricyclic antidepressant	An older class of antidepressant medication that affects serotonin, norepinephrine, and histamine pathways.
Trigeminal neuralgia	A neurologic condition characterized by bouts of severe facial pain.
Trileptal	Brand name for oxcarbazepine, an anticonvulsant medication commonly utilized to treat neuropathic pain.
Tylenol	Brand name for over-the-counter acetaminophen, an analgesic that does not reduce inflammation.
Ultracet	Brand name for a combination of acetaminophen and tramadol, which is a short-acting narcotic-like medication.
Ultram	Brand name for tramadol, a short-acting narcotic-like medication.
UltramER	Brand name for tramadol in a long-acting, once-daily formulation.
Ultrasound	A procedure in which sound waves are generated from a machine, placed over a body part, and then converted into an image of the body.
Valdecoxib	A COX-2 nonsteroidal anti-inflammatory drug that has been removed from the market.
Valium	Brand name for diazepam, a sedating medication commonly used to treat spasticity, muscle spasm, and anxiety.

Valproic acid	An anticonvulsant medication that is commonly used to treat headache, and occasionally used to treat neuropathic pain.
Venlafaxine	A serotonin-norepinephrine reuptake inhibitor antidepressant medication.
Vertebral body	The large cylinder-shaped bone that forms the essential backbone of the spine. There are 7 cervical, 12 thoracic, and 5 lumbar vertebral bodies.
Vicodin	Brand name for a combination of acetaminophen and hydrocodone, which is a short-acting narcotic analgesic medication.
Vicoprofen	Brand name for a combination of ibuprofen and hydrocodone, which is a short-acting narcotic analgesic medication.
Vioxx	Brand name for rofecoxib, a COX-2 nonsteroidal anti-inflammatory drug that has been removed from the market.
Voltaren	Brand name for diclofenac, a nonsteroidal anti-inflammatory drug.
Warfarin	An anticoagulant medication.
Wellbutrin	Brand name for bupropion, an antidepressant medication that blocks the reuptake of dopamine and norepinephrine.
Wholistic medicine	Wholistic medicine views the patient as a whole person, and not simply as a disease or collection of symptoms. Treatment often addresses the multiple dimensions of the individual's physical, emotional, mental and spiritual life. Wholistic medical clinicians usually combine conventional medicine with complementary and alternative medicine, and such an approach is also referred to as "integrative medicine."
X-ray (radiograph)	An image of the body that is obtained by interpreting energy patterns in a specialized plate that is placed behind the patient, who is exposed to radiation energy.

Zanaflex   Brand name for tizanidine, which is a medication that reduces spasticity and acts as a muscle relaxant.

Zoloft   Brand name for sertraline, a serotonin-specific reuptake inhibitor antidepressant medication.

Zonegran   Brand name for zonisamide, an anticonvulsant medication that is sometimes utilized to treat neuropathic pain.

Zonisamide   An anticonvulsant medication that is sometimes utilized to treat neuropathic pain.

Index

Note: Italic *t* indicates a table. Boldface numbers indicate an illustration.